Strength Training for Women at any Age

Gaining Strength During All Stages of Life

Elrey

Table of Contents

We must be willing to get rid of

the life we've planned, so as to have

the life that is waiting for us.

The old skin has to be shed

before the new one can come.

If we fix on the old, we get stuck.

When we hang onto any form,

we are in danger of putrefaction.

Hell is life drying up

—Joseph Campbell

Introduction

Movement is the final common pathway. –C.S. Sherrington

Take out your smartphone. Google Tia-Claire Toomey. If you don't know who Tia is, that's ok. She is only considered The Fittest Woman in the World. She has held the title for five years and is looking good to earn her sixth title. Now go into images. Is this where your mind goes when you think of women who pick up weights? If yes, you are in sympathetic company. If not, then you are among the few. A lot of women find weights intimidating, and their mind goes to the extreme case, i.e., Tia, who is a professional athlete. Tia works out for a living; she has three or four training sessions per day. That is not us. Average women, like you and me, don't have to concern ourselves with getting that 'big.' Because of genetics, even if most of us trained as much as she does, not to mention eat as much as she does, we won't get to that size.

Now that we have gotten that misconception out of the way, there is another one I would like to demystify. Strength and hypertrophy are not the same things. A lot of people use those terms interchangeably or use the word strength to describe hypertrophy (muscle growth). But these are two different adaptations and should be approached differently. They are correlated, however, and we'll get into the details later. And because all good things come in threes, the last misconception I would like to address is that muscles are limited to strength. Muscles are involved in everything that we do. Even if I haven't completely allayed your fears, I hope I have at least let your guard down so that we can have you picking up light weights very soon. Our entry point into the content of this book is to focus on the ten different adaptations that you can get from exercise. We'll zero in on strength training and hypertrophy and their benefits. We'll establish protocols on how to go about training for strength and hypertrophy at different ages. Any good exercise regimen has to be paired with an adequate diet; therefore, we dive into the macronutrients and micronutrients of the diet.

Chapter 1:

Getting Fit at Any Age

For people who spend most of their time sitting down at desks, what Nobel prize winner Charles Scott Sherrington said doesn't seem to ring true. But it is. Our brains developed to the size they are for movement. In the movie *Steve Jobs*, Steve Wozniak asks Jobs what he actually does? "You can't write code, you're not an engineer, you're not a designer, you can't put a hammer to a nail. I built the circuit board, the graphical interface was stolen from Xerox Parc, Jef Raskin was the leader of the Mac team before you threw him off his own project. Everything—someone else designed the box! So how come ten times in a day, I read "Steve jobs is a genius." What do you do?" Job replies in typical Job's fashion "I play the orchestra. And you're a good musician, you sit right there, you're the best in your row." The same can be said about human beings. The cheetah sprints, monkeys can swing and climb, tigers are agile, cetaceans are intelligent, orcas can swim really well and fast, horses can run long distances, kangaroos jump, chimps are really strong, falcons can see very well, and eagles can soar at great heights. So you can imagine all the other mammals asking human beings, "Why are you the apex predator?" The human being replies: "I play the orchestra of movement." Human beings are not just able to swim, we can run as well, and due to our intelligence, and the little help of a Boeing 777, we can fly. That is what makes us remarkable. We are able to move in varied ways, and natural selection has always favored the diverse.

Here we are, in the 21st century, with most of those skills lying dormant with us. We are overweight, slow, and easily physically fatigued. We don't hang, crawl, or climb. Even if we manage to run, we run incorrectly. We run on flat surfaces, in straight lines, with our shoulders hunched over, striking with our heels and our arms, not at right angles. So things are just not looking good. We've obviously decided intelligence is the only skill that matters, but what use is intelligence when one fall can land us with a broken hip? Or having children born through cesarean and losing the benefits of natural birth because women's hips are unable to accommodate the head of the fetus. Non-artificial intelligence, like every other skill, is embodied. The body cannot be dispensed with. We jeopardize this intelligence when they are housed in frail bodies, and once the body decays and dies, so does the intelligence. Aaron Alexander invokes a Joseph Campbell saying with regards to movement: we are "standing on a whale, fishing for minnow." Everything that we need with regards to living in a healthier, stronger, and aligned body is all within our grasp. You are sitting on a gold mine of vitality and health.

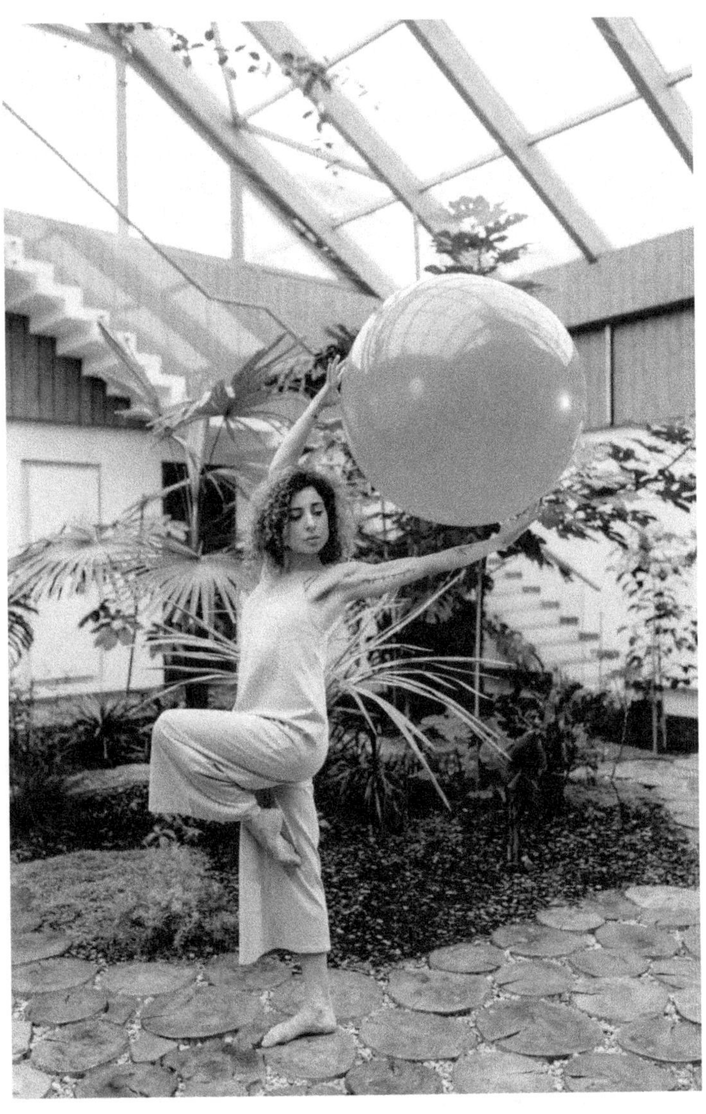

Cliff Booth, pexels.com

Movement

Kelly Starrett, a Doctor of Physical and a trainer, writes in the foreword of *The Align Method*, "What I can tell you with 100 percent certainty is that a few pieces of information apply to you:

1. You have no idea of the depth of your physical capacities or resilience.

2. The resting state of the human is pain-free.

3. Your body is designed to function well over a lifetime that could easily last a hundred years." (Alexander, 2019)

This triptych of information is the tenets of this book. I am going to show you that you are capable of moving in different ways and stretching in different directions, carrying loads you thought you wouldn't be able to and still be strong well into your 80s. We've accepted chronic pain as part of our lives. Pain is information, and the body will keep trying to get your attention through pain. Being in tune with your body will assist you in knowing what to do and how to return your body to a pain-free state. Our bodies have the potential to carry us across a century of living, but we need to remain connected to them. In the psychology sphere, we are told that the body keeps the score. I completely agree, and while this is usually pointing to a demerit system and all the bad things you do to your body or mental well-being, it works in the other direction as well. Your body will keep score of all the good things you do to your body or for your body. "Your vitality is determined by far more than overpriced supplements, complex dietary dogmas, or the latest fitness trends. The way you move impacts every aspect of your life and can be leveraged to make you feel stronger, more confident, and at home in your body." (Alexander, 2019)

"We are coming to realize that the first principles of being human aren't really that complicated or even that sexy: sleep, play, get out in sunlight, eat whole food, foster community, be active in nature, and, perhaps most important, move. Wash, rinse, repeat for the rest of your life." (Alexander, 2019). Alexander touches on something in us that is primal and primordial, which is play. The means we use to express ourselves through movements in our bodies do not have to be completely regimented. Play with your fitness.

Ten Adaptations of Exercise

There are 10 adaptations that you can get from exercise.

- skill
- speed
- power
- strength
- hypertrophy
- muscular endurance
- anaerobic power
- VO2 max

- long duration endurance
- flexibility

Included in the skill adaptation are agility (the ability to change directions very quickly), balance (the ability to distribute weight and remain stable), coordination (the synchronization of moving parts), reaction time (a measure of the time between stimulus and muscle response) and spatial awareness (proprioception which I go into further in the book).

Speed refers to how fast you can do the exercise. Strength is the ability to exert a force. It is generally measured as your one-repetition max. It is a measure of how much weight you can lift if you only had to do it once. Power is the ability to exert a force at a higher speed. In the fitness world, power is defined as explosive strength. Technically, however, power is defined as the rate of doing work. Work is the measure of a force across a distance. Power can also be calculated as the product of the force and the velocity at which that force is applied, i.e., explosive strength. When you are lifting upwards, this is positive work because you are moving the dumbbell upward. As you lower the dumbbell down, you are producing negative work. Negative work just means that the work is being done on the muscle and positive work means that the muscle is doing the work. While you exercise, you and gravity take turns producing work. How quickly you perform your repetitions determines how much power you produce. You want to be able to exert a force at a large enough velocity to be able to overcome gravity.

Endurance is a type of cardiovascular activity which measures the ability to be able to take in oxygen into the body and circulate it within blood across the body. It enables the body to pump a larger volume of blood with each beat. Marathons are an example of long-duration endurance. Muscular endurance is the ability to contract a muscle for long periods of time. When you sprint or go to a spinning class, then you are engaging in cardiovascular activity that is at or near VO2 max.

The degree of movement that occurs at a joint is called the range of motion (ROM). Flexibility is a measure of ROM and has static and dynamic components. There is static and dynamic flexibility. Static flexibility is the range of possible movement about a joint and its surrounding muscles during a passive movement. Static flexibility requires no voluntary muscular activity; an external force such as gravity, a partner, or a machine provides the force for a stretch. Dynamic flexibility refers to the available ROM during active movements and therefore requires voluntary muscular actions. Dynamic ROM is generally greater than static ROM. In yoga, both seem to be important, but there is an order. You start with dynamic flexibility and then move into static flexibility. Static flexibility is effective only once dynamic flexibility has lubricated the joints and warmed the body and muscles.

The Principles of Exercise

There are five principles that you need to always keep at the forefront of your mind whenever you exercise, or else you may be frustrated when the outputs are not what you thought they would be.

The Principle of Adaptations

Exercises themselves do not determine adaptations. The adaptation you require is dependent on other modifiable variables. How those variables are combined will prescribe the change outcomes. The six modifiable variables are exercise choice, intensity, volume, rest, progression, and frequency.

There are no good or bad exercises; there are bad applications. Let's take a goblet squat with dumbbells. Perhaps, you are still a beginner in your training, so there are a few errors you could make. The three main things to consider are complexity, volume, and intensity. Let's look at complexity. A squat is a compound movement, so there are a lot of pieces to maintain form. Perhaps you can't squat low enough (lack of mobility), can't see your toes, and can't keep your back upwards. There are too many pieces, so the recommendation is to use the Smith machines or practice squats without any weights. Other application mistakes could mean that your dumbbell is too heavy for you, so you would have to use a lighter dumbbell or not use one at all. Perhaps you are doing too few repetitions for your desired adaptation or too many.

When it comes to exercises, the default is all joints in full range of motion while maintaining good form.

The Principle of Progressive Overload

Adaptations happens as a product of stress. The principle of overload states that the only way an adaptation can take place is when you increase the volume or intensity of a workout over time. If you stress your body in the same way every day then your body will adjust and adapt and you will no longer see any progress in your training. You have to demand more and more from your body. But you need to be able to rest and recover during and post workouts or else you will not be able to progress. Muscle synthesis happens during rest.

The Principle of Specificity

I'll let Olga Ronnberg, who wrote "Strength Training for Women", write on this principle. "You are good at what you do! If you want more defined muscles but you're dancing in a Zumba class, what do you think is going to happen? I have nothing against Zumba, but do you think you can achieve what you want by dancing? What I'm trying to say is that you have to match your workout to your ultimate goal... Consider attending a Zumba class as your reward and not your main workout." (Ronnberg, 2017).

The Principle of Use/Disuse

This is probably the most sobering of the principles. When you exercise, you make progress and when you stop exercising then you go back to where you were. This book is written across the life of women because exercise has to be seen and experienced through a lifestyle lens. It is not something you can see as a three months goal then you go back to your old ways. Even maintaining progress requires effort. Fall in love with exercise, marry it, and have a "til death do us part" attitude to it.

The Principle of Individual Differences

"One size does not fit all". People are different and uniquely respond to exercises. This is depending on so many factors with genetics probably playing the biggest role in determining these individual differences.

Exercise Across the Different Decades

Women of different ages should all exercise regularly, and although this book is about strength, the different ages of women should supplement their strength training. (Stanfield, 2019)

The 20s:

The goal is to implement healthy habits that will decrease your risk of cardiovascular disease later in life. When you are 20, you could take your youth for granted and therefore not prioritize exercise and eating well. There is a study that was released by the Coronary Artery Risk Development in Young Adults (CARDIA) where they followed 3000 subjects in their twenties. The study revealed that women who had high scores in physical activity coupled with other healthy behaviors such as eating well, very little drinking, if any, and no smoking have a noteworthy lower cardiovascular disease risk profile when they get into middle age.

The 30s:

The goal of this decade is to focus on physical activities that prioritize bone health. According to the National Institute of Health for Osteoporosis and Related Bone Disease National Resource Center, women get osteoporosis in their 50s. We want to move that time further and further away. Osteoporosis is diagnosed later in life, but the process of BMD loss begins earlier. We reach our peak bone mass in the 30s. The formation of bone becomes smaller than bone resorption. The demineralization of bone is resorption. Load-bearing exercises are prioritized to build and maintain bone health. Include resistance training in your workout if you want to go heavier on the weights. Choose aerobic activities that incorporate a load-bearing factor to them, such as a Stairmaster or Zumba. Spinning or swimming is really good aerobically but will not help you to build strong bones. These are very low-impact. On the other side, high-impact aerobic exercises such as tennis or jogging should be included.

Increase your load and intensity over time to improve your bone health and muscular fitness.

The 40s:

The goal of this decade is to prevent age-related muscle loss. Around the age of 40, you start losing muscle mass and strength, and every decade thereafter, it decreases at a rate of 5 lbs per decade. This decline will lead to unwanted weight gain and reduced functional capacity, and you start having muscle imbalances that may cause lower back pain. A study examined recreational athletes who worked out four to five days a week (NCSA, 2015). They were between the ages of 40 and 81 years. The study revealed there was no muscle mass and strength loss. Your muscles atrophy with lack of use, and you can still remain strong into old age.

The 50s:

The goal in this decade is to maintain optimal health as you go through menopause. In the United States, more people die of cardiovascular disease than anything else. After menopause, women, in particular, are at a higher risk of having a heart attack or developing heart disease. This is due to the decrease in estrogen levels. A lot of women's physical activity tapers off during menopause, but an effort should be made to maintain an active lifestyle. Exercise can also help to ease some of the symptoms of menopause.

The 60s:

The goal for this decade is for you to keep moving to prevent falls. A quarter of people over the age of 65 experience a fall annually. Women fall more than men. As you get older, your awareness of your body in space loses acuity. Your reaction time decreases, and a trip can't be prevented from becoming a fall most of the time. Balance training should be included in exercise programs.

The 70s, 80s, and beyond:

The goal is to remember that it is not too late to start exercising. Exercise at this time can help increase your functional capacity. The disability threshold is reached in the late 70s and late 80s. This is the point when you aren't able to perform daily functional activities such as taking a bath and dressing. An active lifestyle will delay the threshold. Functional exercises are emphasized at this time.

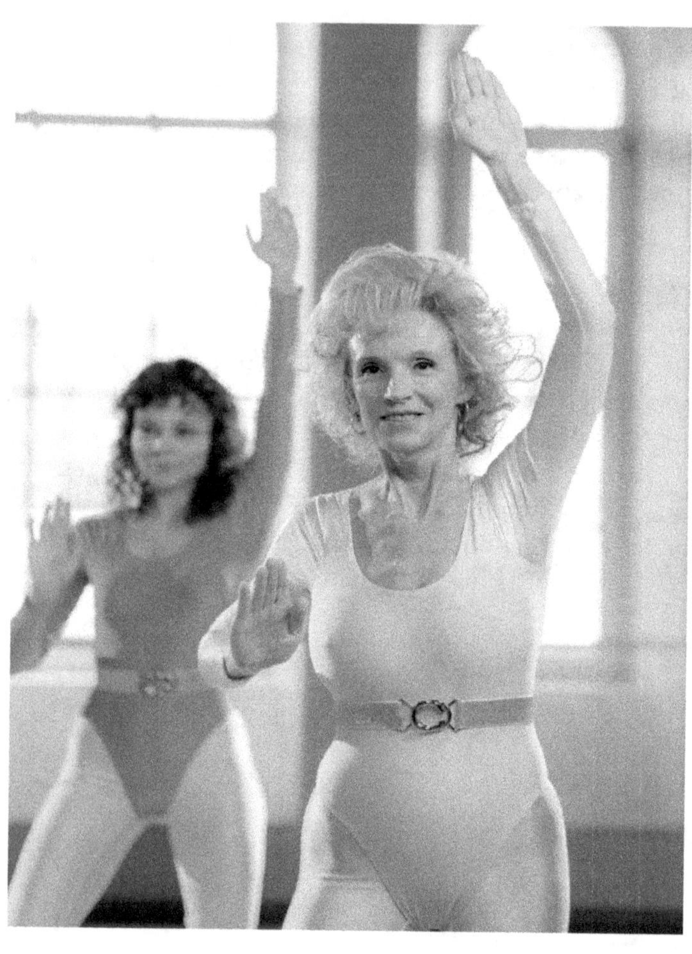

Ron Lach, pexels.com

Chapter 2:

Strength Training

Let's parse the difference between resistance training, weight training, and strength training. Resistance training refers to any type of exercise that causes muscles to contract against external resistance. The main tool used in resistance training is weights. Other tools include your own body weight, rubber or elastic bands, cables, water, hydraulics, or even a vibration platform. Weight training is a form of resistance training where weights are used. Any form of resistance training that enhances muscle strength is strength training.

Bodybuilding is considered an art of building rather than a sport. The primary goal of bodybuilding is to maximize muscle growth (hypertrophy) and, at the same time, decrease body fat. This enhances the sculpting of the body. Any gain in strength is a byproduct and not the main driver.

Weightlifting is an Olympic sport that features two lifts: the snatch and the clean and jerk. These lifts are very technical and are executed explosively and powerfully. Weightlifters are considered the most powerful athletes at the games. Powerlifting touches on skill, speed, power, strength, and flexibility. The snatch and the clean and jerk are used outside of the sport in general strength training because it has the ability to enhance people's power.

The holy trinity of powerlifting is the squat, bench press, and deadlift. While weightlifting enhances power, powerlifting requires pure strength. This is because the lifts are executed with extraordinarily heavy weights that are moved slowly. Elite powerlifters are considered the strongest athletes in the world.

Musculoskeletal System

The musculoskeletal system is made up of joints, tendons, bones, and muscles. These are arranged such that the human body can articulate as many movements as possible. The muscles of the body do not exert a force directly onto an object or onto the ground. Instead, muscles pull against bones, and these bones, which rotate around joints, transmit forces externally. The system of bones allows muscles to be manipulated to produce either a pushing or pulling force against objects in the external environment. In general, without this bone system, muscles can only pull.

Strength training "increases muscular strength, cardiovascular endurance, blood circulation, fat burning, maximal oxygen uptake, lowers blood pressure, improves metabolism, strengthens the skeleton, improves sleep, and reduces the risk for cardiovascular disease." (Ronnberg, 2017)

Hypertrophy

When the muscle's size increases in circumference, this is called hypertrophy. There is a positive correlation between muscle size and muscle strength. However, you can have big muscles without being as strong as your muscles would lead everyone to believe. For example, let's take those machines that you press against your abdomen, and your abdomen muscles grow and become "six-pack abs." Technically, you have a six-pack, but you are not strong because your core is weak. The number one exercise that makes your core stronger but doesn't really make your abs show is the plank. This is just an illustration that just because you have the muscles.

It doesn't mean that you are strong. Let me clarify that you can be both, which is the reason that there is a positive relationship between the two. There are mechanical and metabolic factors that play a role in the optimization of muscle growth. The inclusion of eccentric muscle actions, heavy load limiting, and low to moderate volumes are the mechanical factors that are also in strength training. Metabolic factors are focused on intensity that is low- to moderate, or high when they are executed in conjunction with high volumes.

Bone size can be increased if the exercises that you are doing are above the Minimal Essential Strain (MES). This is the threshold that has to be crossed in order for bone formation to occur. The exercises have to be progressive so that the forces that are generated exceed the MES in order to facilitate bone size and strength.

The bones have to increase in size and strength to be able to support larger and larger loads. An increase in muscle mass and strength increases bone mineral density (BMD). The BMD is the amount of mineral that is deposited in a certain part of the bone. When you do not work out at all, your bones lose density very quickly. People who work out with resistance have a higher BMD than their peers who do not work out. Therefore, exercises that lead to hypertrophy and gains in strength also lead to bone growth. Bone adaptations take place over a long period of time (six months), but the effects start happening with your first few workouts. There are substances that are already being deposited into the bloodstream in the first few workouts. But it's important that you play the long game when it comes to osteogenesis.

The specificity of loading is important when it comes to working out to increase bone strength. You have to load the bones that you are trying to strengthen. When you are trying to develop the bones in your legs, you may sprint, but if you want to develop the bones in your wrists, then you may want to do more gymnastic or calisthenic types of movements. Osteoporosis is a condition that takes place where BMD levels decrease to the point where your bones become brittle, and then you are prone to injuries. You want to engage in structural exercises (exercises that work through the spine and the hip) and involve as many joints as possible. The load has to be heavy enough as well. Machines in the gym are not good for the promotion of osteogenesis because the machine does the job of supporting the body. Free weights promote bone growth because the internal structure has to support the body.

The principle of progressive overload also applies to bone growth. You have to place a load that exceeds the normal demands on the bones. Bones respond to higher forces than those required to maintain bone strength. The bones adapt to become stronger to prevent the risk of stress fractures. Younger bones respond to osteogenic stimulation more than mature bones, so it would make sense to start resistance training as young as possible. Exercising or engaging in other physical activities during growth also has the effect of modeling the structure of the person optimally. Peak bone mass is elevated when you are younger and contributes positively to bone mass later in life. When the bone undergoes stress and re-forms, it does so in such a way that the collagen fibers anticipate the direction of the load. The load has to be loaded in different directions so that the collagen fibers respond differently and the bone becomes stronger globally. A volume of around 30 to 35 repetitions is sufficient to generate the necessary adaptations. "The components of mechanical load that stimulate bone growth are the magnitude of the load (intensity), rate (speed) of loading, direction of the forces, and the volume of loading (number of repetitions)." (NSCA,2015)

The following summarizes the factors that you need to consider to ensure that you stimulate bone formation.

HOW YOU CAN STIMULATE BONE FORMATION

- Choose multi-joint exercises that target the entire structure.
- Choose exercises that work through the spine and the hips.
- Apply the principle of progressive overload.
- Exercise using heavy loads and exercise using high impact movements (jumping) to expose the bone to different directional stimuli.
- Vary your exercises.

All connective tissue (tissue that joins bones and muscles) is the collagen fiber. In bone, ligaments, and tendons, it is Type I, and for cartilage, it is Type II. Tendons do not get a lot of oxygen and therefore take a lot of time to heal from injury. Ligaments need to be able to stretch in order to accommodate the range of motion of joints. Tendons and ligaments attach to bone and it's their attachment strength that allows for maximum force transmission. Anaerobic exercise consistently executed can lead to connective tissue adaptations. As you get stronger and as your muscles get bigger, your connective tissue has to also adapt for strength and muscle growth. Connective tissue can get stronger where they are able to carry loads: the place where the tendon and ligament meet bone, within the tendon or ligament, and in the skeletal muscle (fascia). Resistance training increases the amount of collagen in the connective tissue. The critical factor in maximizing tendon stiffness is the intensity of exercise. Cartilage provides smooth movement of joints, acts as a shock absorber for forces on the joint, and assists in how connective tissue attaches to the bone. Oxygen also takes a while to reach cartilage which means it takes a long time to repair as well. Cartilage gets oxygen as the joint moves. If the joint does not move, cells die because they don't get the nutrients and oxygen they need. Genetics plays a big role in how cartilage responds to stimuli.

Benefits of Strength Training

The following table (NSCA, 2015) is a summary of what happens in the body when you work out using resistance. These adaptations are not comprehensive; only those that are relevant have been included. These adaptations, collectively, improve performance in strength, power, and muscular endurance.

PHYSIOLOGICAL ADAPTATIONS TO RESISTANCE TRAINING	
Performance:	
• Muscle strength	Increases
• Muscle endurance	Increases with a high-power output
• Aerobic power	Negligible

• Anaerobic power	Increases
• Rate of force generation	Increases
• Vertical jump	Improves
• Sprint speed	Improves
• Flexibility	Increases
Muscle Fibers:	
• Cross-sectional area (girth)	Increases
Connective Tissue:	
• Ligament strength	Increase
• Collagen content	Increase
• Tendon strength	Increase
• Bone density	Increase or no change
Body Composition:	
• Body fat %	Decreases
• Lean body mass	Increases
Respiratory and Cardiovascular system	
• Cardiac output	Increases

• Stroke volume	Increases
• Heart rate	Increases
• Oxygen uptake	Increases
• Systolic blood pressure	Increases
• Blood flow	Increases

Factors That Influence Strength Training

Biological and Chronological Age

We all know that people develop very differently. In general, the growth process is marked by milestones, and people hit those milestones at different times; therefore, there are two types of ages that need to be considered. The first is the chronological age which is measured in years and months, and from the day you are born to the day you die, it just keeps on adding. Biological age is more concerned with what's happening internally within you. For example, someone who looks young for their age is someone whose biological age and chronological age do not match. You know, from when you were a young girl, that all of us had menarche at different ages. Some girls sexually matured earlier than others. I myself was what we would call a late bloomer, and I had a growth spurt later in my teens than earlier. So my biological age is younger than my chronological. And because I've been active most of my life and I've been instructing fitness for seven years, I suspect that my biological age is still lagging behind my chronological age. So you can obviously see the downside to this when it comes to sports, usually; we were grouped according to our chronological age rather than our biological age. It was no wonder that the girl who looked older than all of us always won. Measures of fitness are used to measure maturation. Performance of motor skills and strength development are some of the things that are measured. Physical activity, especially those that generate compressive forces, is important for skeletal remodeling and growth. The skeletal age assessment is the main assessment used to determine biological age.

Training Age

People are living longer and there are also more older people who are even participating in sports like marathon running. After the age of thirty, a lot of people experience a decline in performance until age 70, when it decreases even more dramatically. Older people who do not engage in physical activities see a rise in debilitating injuries. It is well known that muscle and bone decrease with age. This doesn't just make it difficult to do simple things like sit in a chair or open a window, but there is the risk of a fall or fracture that can lead to long-term disability. Bones become more porous as they lose BMD. The hip, spine, or wrist are particularly vulnerable. Osteopenia is a measure of

BMD loss. In a more aggravated form, it becomes osteoporosis. Women are more likely to get injured than men.

Factors that contribute to BMD loss include physical inactivity, hormones, nutrition, and genetics. Sarcopenia is the term given to the loss of muscle mass and strength. After the age of 30, there is a decrease in muscle density, tendon compliance, and an increase in muscle fat. Women experience these deleterious effects worse than men. Most of this atrophy can be attributed to inactivity. What you don't use, you lose. This loss of muscle mass and strength is a marker of a loss to generate power. Power is required in the execution of everyday activities. Power degenerates even faster than muscle mass and strength. Power is diminished due to a decrease in muscle mass, changes in the nervous system, hormonal changes, inadequate nutrition, and physical inactivity. Sarcopenia can lead to people becoming functionally dependent on other people or technology to assist them in doing normal daily activities. The following table compares the effects of aging and resistance training on physiology.

PHYSIOLOGICAL CHANGES TO AGE AND RESISTANCE TRAINING		
	AGE	**RESISTANCE TRAINING**
Strength	Decreases	Increases
Power	Decreases	Increases

Endurance	Decreases	Increases
Muscle mass	Decreases	Increases
Muscle fiber size	Decreases	Increases
Muscular metabolic capacity	Decreases	Increases
Resting metabolic rate	Decreases	Increases
% Body fat	Increases	Decreases
BMD	Decreases	Increases
Physical functionality	Decreases	Increases

When you are young, a fall is funny, but as you grow older, falls are breath-holding moments where people are really worried about the extent of the damage. When you are older, you don't easily come back intact from a fall. Quality of life decreases because of all the health, economic, and psychosocial consequences that come as a result. A fall can lead to joint dislocations, pain, skeletal fractures, and the inability to carry out daily functional activities. People's self-confidence also takes a hit. A fall can also result in institutionalization or, even worse, result in a fatality. A decrease in muscle strength and power combined with a slow reaction time, impaired balance, and postural instability lead to falls being dangerous. When you fall, your body generally anticipates the hit with the ground, and a shock absorbing effect takes place. The joint is stabilized through a motor control strategy called cocontraction. Preactivation takes place as you are falling, and the limbs stiffen and are able to come in contact with the ground without breaking anything. Older people need to exercise in such a way that they are able to have a more strategic relationship with gravity and the floor. When it comes to seniors, exercise is just not enough. You want to incorporate exercises that increase balance, coordination, and reaction time.

Resistance training by itself would not be able to prevent falls. The good news is that "aging does not appear to enhance or reduce the ability of the musculoskeletal system to adapt to resistance exercise. Significant improvements in muscular strength, muscular power, muscle mass, bone mineral density, and functional capabilities (e.g., gait speed) have been observed in older people who participated in progressive resistance training programs. For older adults, such improvements enhance exercise performance, decrease the risk of injury, promote independent living, and improve quality of life." (NSCA, 2015). When older people start exercising, their medical history plays a huge role in how the exercise program looks. Safety becomes even more critical because the margins of error are very small for older people. The safety recommendations for resistance training for older people are listed in the following table.

RESISTANCE TRAINING SAFETY PRECAUTIONS FOR OLDER ADULTS

- Older adults should be screened before undertaking any resistance training because they usually suffer from age-related medical conditions.

- There should be a 5–10 minute low—to moderate—warm-up before every exercise session.

- Static stretching is paramount to increasing their mobility and should take place before or after the exercise session.

- The resistance training used must not be too excessive.

- They should not perform the Valsalva maneuver at all.

- There should be a recovery period of 48 to 72 hours.

- Any pain in joints should be avoided.

In addition to exercise, older people must eat more high-quality protein. To not eat well is to expose yourself to the loss of bone mass and strength and to expose yourself to fatigue, a compromised immune system, and extended recovery time.

Gender

Gender plays an important role in how people adapt to exercise stimuli. "Women who regularly participate in resistance training activities can improve their health, reduce their risk of degenerative diseases (e.g., osteoporosis) and their injury rates, and enhance their overall sporting performance. Whereas in the past, women may have questioned the value of resistance training or even avoided this type of exercise due to social stigma, evidence clearly indicates that women are capable of tolerating and adapting to the stresses of resistance exercise and that the benefits are substantial. Furthermore, to enhance health and fitness and reduce injury rates, it is now suggested that resistance training be an essential component of any training program that females follow." (NSCA, 2015)

Prepubescent girls and boys show no marked differences in weight, height, or body size. Puberty brings substantial changes and marked differences between boys and girls, mainly because of the different hormones being released into the bodies. Estrogen in young girls increases the fat deposits around the body, including breast development, and testosterone in young boys increases how their bones form and how protein is synthesized. Adult males have a greater structure than women because males have a longer growth period than women. Estrogen does produce bone growth, but the shorter growth period limits the amount of bone growth. In comparison to their male counterparts, women have more body fat, smaller muscles, and less bone mineral density. Women are also lighter in mass compared to men. The fact that men have a larger frame means that they can support more muscle tissue than women's structures can.

There are two measures when it comes to how women and men respond to muscular strength: relative and absolute strength. The lower body of women and the lower body of men have very close absolute strengths in comparison to each other. However, when it comes to the upper body, women have fewer muscles than men, in the absolute sense. On a relative basis, differences in muscular strength based on sex are drastically less.

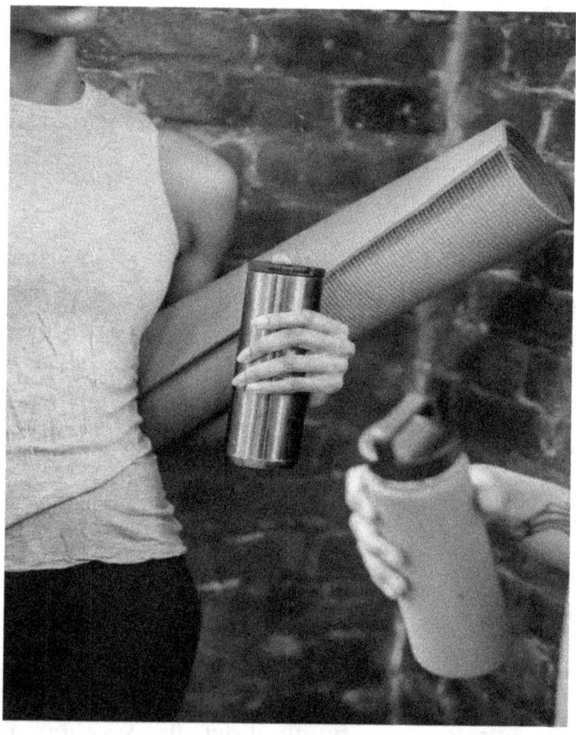

Klaus Nielsen, pexels.com

The average man and woman differ with regards to lean body mass, strength relative to body weight, and the size of muscles. The relative strength of men and women is similar when looking at lean body mass.

However, relative strength to body weight for men is still higher than for women. Eccentric strength is similar for women and men, and the differences widen when you move to concentric strength. Muscle quality is not sex-dependent. What this means is that there is a direct relationship between the size of muscle and strength, irrespective of sex. The muscle fibers and type are the same for men and women. Because of individual differences, two women may show even more differences than a man and a woman.

Men and women respond to resistance training in the same way. The magnitudes will be different, but the overall adaptation will be the same. Women can increase their strength at a faster rate in comparison to males, or it can be at the same rate. Hypertrophy is not just limited to men; women can also experience that adaptation if they work out regularly with high intensity or high volume. Testosterone levels in women vary and women who have higher levels of testosterone are able to increase their muscle size more easily than women who have lower levels of testosterone. There are women who are genetically predisposed to develop larger muscles than other women.

In athletics, there is a term called Female Athlete Triad, which needs to be considered in order to ensure that the woman does not suffer any negative health outcomes while training strength and conditioning. The triad describes the interplay between a women's menstrual function, her energy availability, and bone mineral density. When women train for longer periods, and they do not consume enough calories to supply the necessary energy to achieve their adaptations, it is a health risk. Osteoporosis is likely to occur when women do not eat enough. Amenorrhea, the condition where a menstrual cycle is absent for three months or more, can take place. The effects of amenorrhea on women include bone stress fractures, hormonal complications, gastrointestinal complications, and a decrease in performance.

Resistance exercises mitigate age-related BMD declines. In fact, it can even serve to increase bone mass and structural remodeling. Higher intensities of resistance exercises will produce an onset of osteogenesis. Women should start resistance training while younger (preadolescents) to set their BMD up for the future. Your nutritional intake has to be sufficient to make sure that those adaptations actually take place and you recover properly. Women are more likely to suffer from body dysmorphia because of pressures to look a certain way, and they may not eat enough as a result. This will end with them suffering the consequences of the Female Athlete Triad.

There is no difference in the resistance training programs for women and for men because the same muscles are being targeted. The difference will come in with regards to the loads, but the adaptations will be the same. Younger women must train resistance training to ensure that when they become adults, they have tapped into their maximum musculoskeletal potential. Women should focus on working out the upper body to improve their upper body strength. Sometimes the fact that the upper body is underdeveloped may lead to underperformance in multi-joint exercises, which are important in strength training. Women are more susceptible to knee injuries than men are. The contributing factors are: uncontrolled joint movements, misalignment in limbs, body movements that do not adhere to correct form, poor technique, hormonal changes, and an unconducive shoe-surface interaction. The risk of ACL injury is higher for women because their musculature doesn't really develop fully. Training these muscles in youth will strengthen the ACL. Exercises should include resistance training, plyometrics (jumping), and agility (ability to change direction quickly and correctly). Knee injuries happen when women land (eccentric loading) and pivot laterally. In conjunction with a good training program, women should ensure that they eat enough high-quality protein and good fats that are needed to get adaptations.

Heredity

"Body type, or somatotype, refers to the idea that there are three generalized body compositions that people are predetermined to have. The concept was theorized by Dr. W.H. Sheldon back in the early 1940s, naming the three somatotypes endomorph, mesomorph, and ectomorph. It was originally believed that a person's somatotype was unchangeable and that certain physiological and psychological characteristics were even determined by whichever one a person aligns to. According to Sheldon, endomorphs have bodies that are always rounded and soft, mesomorphs are always square and muscular, and ectomorphs are always thin and fine-boned. He theorized that these body types directly influenced a person's personality, and the names were chosen because he believed the predominant traits of each somatotype were set in stone, derived from pre-birth preferential development of either the endodermal, mesodermal, or ectodermal embryonic layers." (Payen, 2022)

Although Sheldon was incorrect in his conclusions, he was correct in his initial assumptions. There are three main body types, but they are not set in stone and can change. Sheldon had it backward; he believed that our somatotype determined our physiology, but it is our physiology that determines our current somatotype. "No one exists within purely one somatotype; instead, we are all constantly in flux and fall uniquely on a spectrum between all three... As they are understood and accepted today, body types reflect a generalized picture of how a person's physiology is functioning in their current state. The observable somatotype represents the current sum of their physical, dietary, and lifestyle choices up to that point in time, combined with a variety of uncontrollable factors influenced by both genetics and the surrounding environment." (Payne, 2022). The different somatotypes are described in the following table by focusing on metabolism, structure, and how fat is deposited in the body.

SOMATOTYPES		
ENDOMORPH	**MESOMORPH**	**ECTOMORPH**
• stockier bone structures with large hips and midsection • more fat throughout the body • gains fat quickly and loses it slowly • slow metabolism usually because of an inactive lifestyle and daily calorific surplus	• shoulders wider than hips and a medium frame • athletic musculature • efficient metabolism, gain and lose mass very easily	• narrow hips and shoulders relative to height • smaller muscles relative to bone length • naturally fast metabolism which makes it difficult to gain mass • if BMI is less than 17, indicative of an eating disorder

Chapter 3:

Training Physiology

We are about to get super technical in this chapter, and we go into the nitty and gritty parts of your bodies. This is important because it will empower you. You will understand why perhaps you like certain exercises more than others and why training certain muscles are hard. You will even understand how energy travels in your system and fuels your workouts. You will understand different types of exercise in detail and know how adaptations show themselves in your body and how you perform or move. Your body is a hormetic system that can alert you to things it may need through inflammation or stress. You will better understand what lactate does in your body and how you can work out such that even when you are done with your workout, your body is still burning calories. Let's start with the muscle fibers and muscle actions.

Muscle Fibers

Motor neurons transmit electrochemical impulses from the spinal cord to the muscle, which innervate muscle fibers. A motor neuron is usually able to activate different muscle fibers. I've included a bit of this technical detail so that you understand the different muscle types because fundamentally, the neuromuscular system determines the muscle fiber type and its function, characteristics, and how it's recruited and utilized during exercise. The impulse that is fired by a motor neuron is called the action potential. When an action potential is released, all the fibers that the motor neuron serves are activated at the same time, and a force is developed. The number of muscle fibers within each motor unit will prescribe how much control a muscle has. For example, the eye, which functions with high precision, may even have a one-to-one relationship between a motor neuron and muscle fiber, whereas a big muscle such as your hamstring is less precise. Therefore, one motor neuron can activate hundreds of muscle fibers. Any change in the number of motor units that are active can produce disproportionally high changes in the acuity of the force that needs to move the eye in a precise way. The electric current (action potential) is not able to activate a muscle fiber directly; instead, the current causes the release of a chemical that activates the muscle fiber. Once enough chemicals have been released, the muscle contracts. All of the muscle fibers of that motor unit simultaneously contract, and a force in the muscle is developed simultaneously as well.

A twitch occurs when the muscle contracts briefly. This brief contraction results from an action potential making its way to motor neurons and activating muscle fibers. When the muscle fiber is activated, calcium is released within the fiber, and a force generates. Before the force generates to its maximum, the calcium is removed from the fiber, and the muscle relaxes. If a second twitch is produced from the motor neuron before the muscle fully relaxes, then two twitches coincide, and the force that is produced is bigger than the force produced when only one twitch was produced. Therefore, the less time between twitches, the higher the force generated within muscle fibers. Tetanus is the condition that occurs when the duration between twitches decreases so much that the twitches fuse. Tetanus is the maximum amount of force that can be produced by the motor unit.

The fibers of skeletal muscles are classified according to their twitch time: Slow-twitch and fast-twitch. Fast-twitch fibers contract and relax very quickly and have a short switch time. Slow-twitch fibers, however, develop force and relax slowly with a lengthy twitch time. These fibers have different physiological and morphological characteristics. These fibers can also be classified as Type I and Type II, which are slow-twitch and fast-twitch, respectively. Mechanically, their biggest distinction lies in the ability to meet the energy demands of the muscle fiber, which consequently affects the ability of the fiber to withstand fatigue. Type I fibers are generally able to withstand fatigue, are efficient, and capable of a high capacity for the supply of aerobic energy. The drawback of Type I fibers is that they have a limited ability to generate force rapidly. Type II is the opposite of Type I—they are inefficient, easily fatigable, and have a high capacity for anaerobic energy supply. Postural muscles are mostly composed of Type I fibers, while large muscles used to locomote have a combination of Type 1 and Type II so that both low (jogging) and high (sprinting) power output activities can be executed.

A muscle force output is dependent on the task at hand. We know that movement is divided into gross motor skills and fine motor skills. When you move your hand, you are making use of fine motor skills, which are smooth and coordinated. When you jump, you are making use of gross motor skills. Your muscles match force output to the task so that you can pick a pencil off the floor. Too much force output lands you with a broken pencil or a broken finger, or you just will not be able to coordinate the movement enough to pick up the pencil. The higher the frequency that individual motor units fire, the higher the force output of the whole muscle. There is another way to increase the force output of a muscle apart from increasing the frequency. This process is called recruitment, and in this case, more motor units fire. Okay, that was a lot of technical information, but it was important to establish the fundamentals of movement. The following table is a summary of different sports and which muscle fibers are involved.

RELATIVE INVOLVEMENT OF MUSCLE FIBER TYPES IN SPORTS EVENTS

	TYPE I	TYPE II
100 m sprint	Low	High
800 m run	High	High
Marathon	High	Low
Olympic weightlifting	Low	High
Soccer, lacrosse, hockey	High	High
Basketball, netball	Low	High
Boxing	High	High
50 m swim	Low	High
Field events	Low	High
Cross-country skiing, biathlon	High	High
Tennis	High	High
Speed skating	High	High
Track cycling	Low	High
Rowing	High	High

| Wrestling | High | High |
| Distance cycling | High | Low |

The table can be used to make inferences regarding other exercise activities. Gymnasts are considered amongst the strongest people in sports, and both Type I and Type II are high. Traditional Ashtanga yoga would be high in Type II and low in Type I. A 60-minute power yoga asana practice would make use of more Type I muscle fibers than Type II. A combination of the two would recruit both types of muscle fibers. Spinning and Zumba would recruit both.

The force that a muscle can exert corresponds to its cross-sectional area and not its volume. Let's take two gym members who have a similar body fat composition and biceps that have the same circumference, but one of the gym members is tall, and the other is short. The taller member has a larger volume of muscle but produces the same force as the short one because they have the same circumference. This means that they produce the same force, but the shorter member is able to get a better outcome because they have a less gravitational force to overcome than the taller and heavier member. If you want to increase the strength of a muscle, you have to increase its cross-sectional area and, therefore, its circumference.

Muscle Action

There are three different muscle actions: concentric, eccentric, and isometric action. In concentric muscle action, the muscle shortens, and in eccentric muscle actions, the muscle lengthens. The risk of soreness or injury increases with eccentric movements because the force that the muscle produces is less than the external forces to stretch the tendon. In isometric muscle action, the forces generated internally and externally are equal. Take a bicep curl with a dumbbell. When you lift the dumbbell up towards the shoulders, then the muscle action is concentric, and when you lower the dumbbell down, it's eccentric. Isometric action happens when you hold the dumbbell in your hand with your forearms perpendicular to the upper arm at the elbow. This is called an isometric hold.

Bioenergetics

There are two types of exercise-related bioenergetics that we will discuss: aerobic and anaerobic metabolism. Aerobic exercises can only be executed in the presence of oxygen, whereas anaerobic exercises do not require oxygen. Only carbohydrates (of the three macronutrients) can be metabolized for energy without oxygen being present. If you are going to be doing anaerobic exercises, then carbohydrates are critical. Anaerobic exercises include resistance training, and aerobic exercises are running and swimming. Fat can be used as a fuel, but it takes a much longer time to be used than carbohydrates.

Lactate

When you work out very hard and start feeling the so-called burn, then there is lactate present. A lot of people incorrectly call this lactic acid, but that is not produced by human beings. As we increase the intensity or volume of a workout, we make our way towards the anaerobic threshold. This means that once we feel the burn, our body needs oxygen. Do not stop working out. Lactate is not a signal that you are pushing yourself too much; it is a signal of lack of oxygen and buffering against acidity in the blood. Lactate itself can act as fuel for you to push through the burn. When you do that, the muscle health of your organs is improved. (Huberman, 2022)

Excess Postexercise Oxygen Consumption

"Most [people] are aware of the high caloric burn that takes place during high-intensity cardiovascular training, such as a Spinning class. However, less commonly known is the fact that a small tweak to the intensity or structure of your workouts can elevate the phenomenon known as excessive post-exercise oxygen consumption (EPOC) for hours after your workouts are over. That extra burn can translate into more total calories burned, additional weight loss benefits, and enhanced performance during each session! EPOC refers to the elevation in metabolism (rate that calories are burned) after an exercise session ends. The increased metabolism is linked to increased consumption of oxygen, which is required to help the body restore and return to its pre-exercise state. (Ward, 2022). The following table summarizes the effect that the different exercises have on EPOC.

EPOC: Intensity, Mode, and Duration

Aerobic Exercise:

- intensity has the largest effect on EPOC

- a high intensity coupled with a high duration produces the highest EPOC

- high-Intensity Interval Training (HIIT) will produce a high EPOC at lower workloads

Resistance Training:

- heavy resistance training will yield a higher EPOC than circuit weight training

- intensity matters

Factors Responsible for EPOC:

- oxygen in blood and muscle is replenished

- resynthesis of the fuel (ATP) in the body

- body temperature, ventilation, and circulation are high

- protein turnover is high

- the body is becoming efficient as it recovers

Interval Training

Interval training allows for a more efficient energy utilization by making use of a work-to-rest ratio that is predetermined. This allows you to increase intensity and get more work done in a shorter period of time. The fatigue levels are less or the same as continuous training at moderate intensity.

High-Intensity Interval Training (HIIT) is a training regimen that alternates between high intensity with rest periods in between. HIIT "is today considered one of the most effective forms of exercise for physical performance in athletes." (NSCA, 2015). There are nine different variables that can be changed and manipulated in order to achieve a specific metabolic outcome:

- mode of exercise
- intensity of the active part of each cycle
- duration of the active part of each cycle
- duration of the recovery part of each cycle
- intensity of the recovery part of each cycle
- number of cycles in a set
- number of sets
- set rest time
- recovery intensity between sets

HIIT provides the same physiological and performance adaptations as endurance training, except that these adaptations are achieved much quicker.

Combination Training

Combination training, also known as cross-training, is when long endurance activities are incorporated into the training regime. When people's aerobic fitness is good, their power output recovery is quicker. Aerobic training may decrease anaerobic capabilities, maximum strength, size of muscles, and power output. This has been traditionally called the interference effect, but there is a lot of contention regarding this, and some scientists believe the amount of volume is so much that it is becoming deleterious. There seems to be an asymmetry about this, however. People who are more aerobically inclined benefit from adding anaerobic activity. It improves their high-intensity endurance performance.

Hormones

Heavy resistance training consistently undertaken over long periods of time improves the trained muscles' size, strength, and power. Hormones are released prior to, during, and post a resistance exercise. The demands of an exercise, the recovery, and the adaptation of the exercise all lead to changes in hormones—these changes signal the tissue to adapt to the exercises. Heavy resistance training increases the amount of testosterone in the muscle. It is the release of testosterone coupled with the tearing and repairing of muscle that increases muscle strength and growth. If the stress on the muscle is too large, the muscles don't repair as they should, and you lose size and strength in the muscle. "Hormone responses are tightly linked to the characteristics of the resistance exercise protocol." (NSCA, 2015). The release of hormones is dependent on the demand of the exercise. If you do light resistance training, your hormones would not respond to this because the base levels are able to meet the demand. Adaptations only occur with stress. If the resistance exercise you are doing is not stressing your body, then there is no adaptation taking place. Hormones are secreted in response to a need for homeostatic control in the body; the endocrine system is part of an overall strategy to bring physiological functions back into normal range. These homeostatic mechanisms controlled by the endocrine system can be activated in response to an acute (immediate) resistance exercise stress or can be altered by chronic (over longer periods of time) resistance training. The mechanism that mediates acute homeostatic changes to acute resistance exercise stress is typically a sharp increase or decrease in hormonal concentrations to regulate a physiological variable, such as glucose level. A more subtle increase or decrease usually occurs in chronic resting hormonal concentrations in response to resistance training. (NSCA, 2015)

Androgens

Testosterone is the main androgen that is associated with muscle tissue. Its presence in the system can signal the release of growth hormone, which can lead to the synthesis of protein. Testosterone does not just influence muscle strength and size but also has an effect on the nervous system. Testosterone that increases during high-intensity aerobic activity is related to the need for protein synthesis. During this type of activity, catabolic (breaking down of muscle) may be taking place. Even if testosterone is increased, this repair is not hypertrophic because aerobic exercises do not make muscles bigger. Testosterone concentrations can be increased through large group muscle exercises, heavy resistance loads, a high volume of exercise, and short rest intervals. The time of day that you exercise does not have an impact on the concentration of testosterone or the increase in strength. Women have much lower levels of testosterone, but they are able to use the testosterone that they already have in resistance training. The response in women is higher than in men.

Women have significantly lower levels of testosterone than men because testosterone is primarily a male sex hormone. The increase in testosterone for women after resistance training is very low. There is an exception, however—young women in their twenties are able to increase their testosterone during resistance training if their volume is very large. Levels of testosterone can actually be variegated between individual women because there are women who produce high levels of testosterone.

Growth Hormone

Growth hormone plays a large role in child development, but it also plays a role in assisting the body to adapt to stress caused by resistance training.

Growth hormone increases the transportation of amino acids across cell membranes, protein synthesis, the breakdown of fat (lipolysis), the synthesis of collagen, the growth of cartilage, and the function of the immune cell. Gender, sleep, age, nutrition, exercise, and alcohol intake affect the release patterns of growth hormones. Growth hormone is released when resistance training is executed at the right intensity. "Growth hormone release is affected by the type of resistance training protocol used including the duration of rest period. Short rest period types of workouts result in greater serum concentrations compared to long rest protocols of similar total work." (NSCA, 2015)

With women, the release of growth hormone varies with the menstrual cycle because the base levels of the hormone are different at different parts of the cycle. Also, women who are on birth control release much higher growth hormone during resistance exercise. Regardless, both women and men show an increase in growth hormone when resistance training takes place with low rest intervals.

Cortisol

Cortisol is the main hormone that signals the use of carbohydrates as fuel. Cortisol is highest in the mornings and tapers as the day proceeds. It stimulates the production of carbohydrates through the conversion of amino acids. When cortisol is present, protein synthesis is inhibited. Cortisol degrades both Type I and Type II muscle fibers, but due to the sheer number of proteins in Type II, cortisol degradates those fibers more. When you are sick or injured, the presence of cortisol causes muscle atrophy, so you lose strength. The cortisol that is released during exercise cause inflammation in the tissue. Resistance exercises consisting of large volumes and small rest intervals cause a large amount of cortisol to be released. When it comes to cortisol, the chronic release of it is catabolic but acute levels of it will cause the muscle tissue to remodel. In the process of becoming stronger, the muscles break down to rebuild again, and cortisol is one of the ways that this process can take place. Cortisol also removes damaged proteins from the muscles.

Catecholamines: Epinephrine, Dopamine, Norepinephrine

People who have higher catecholamines released before and during resistance training are able to have a better workout than if those catecholamines are low. They are able to sustain force throughout the workout. Epinephrine and norepinephrine increase how much force is produced by a muscle, muscle contraction rate, blood pressure, blood flow in muscle, and energy availability.

The following graph summarizes how you can manipulate the endocrine (hormonal) system with resistance training.

MANIPULATING THE ENDOCRINE SYSTEM WITH RESISTANCE TRAINING

General:

- When you use more muscles, then you potentially increase the remodeling of tissue.
- You can only adapt muscles that are targeted during resistance training.

Increase in Testosterone Concentrations:

- Use exercises that target large muscle groups.
- Use heavy resistance.
- Exercise with minimally moderate volumes.
- Have short rest periods.

Increase Growth Hormone Concentrations:

- You want to get lactate to be released; therefore, exercises that are high in intensity should be selected.
- Eat carbohydrates and protein pre and post-workouts.

Optimize Adrenal Hormones:

- Use large muscle groups, high volume, and short rest periods.
- Make sure that you have days of rest so that the adrenals are not overworked, and you don't want cortisol to be released chronically either.

Detraining

Detraining occurs when your body starts losing the adaptations that you have accumulated through a decrease in frequency, intensity, or volume. The principle of reversibility states that whatever strength and muscle growth you have achieved can disappear when the stimulus is no longer there, or it is not enough to maintain those gains. The longer you go without working out, the higher the adaptation losses. There is a lag time between when you stop working out and when the adaptations start to diminish. You will start losing strength after four weeks of continuous inactivity.

Training Physiology Across the Decades

The 20s:

This is the time when your hormone levels are the highest, you have a high libido, and your cognitive ability is super sharp. The mood swings that you had experienced during the preceding decade have diminished substantially. You are prone to joint injury, and there is a high probability of your anterior cruciate tearing. Strengthen your hip and thigh muscles. You are also at your most fertile, and your body is preparing for childbirth. As a result, you have higher flexibility in the back, and you experience more pressure in your lower back. Women in their 20s should look out for polycystic ovarian disease, which may cause a lot of hormonal imbalances. You may experience insulin resistance and gain weight. The high levels of hormones keep the arteries flexible, and heart disease is not a concern for you.

The 30s:

The hormone levels start decreasing. Supplement your diet with folic acid, vitamin D, and Omega 3's. The decline in hormone levels will lead to weight gain. Women gain 3-5 pounds every decade. Your waist grows as fat is deposited there. Unfortunately, you cannot target specific body areas when trying to tackle fat. Include a bit of cardio in your workouts, and fat stores can be targeted. Your BMD experiences a decline, and therefore you need to incorporate weight-bearing exercises in your life. Your skin is beginning to lose its hyaluronic acid. Incorporate yoga into your routine.

The 40s:

This is when women are in perimenopause, and therefore your body is in one of its unpredictable times. Your hormone levels will take a much steeper decline, and they will be very erratic. Your menstruation will be longer and heavier, and sometimes you may miss a month here and there. Rest as much as you need to between exercise sessions and make sure that you eat sufficiently and adequately. You will also experience more fatigue, so your exercise sessions may be limited. Your metabolism also decreases, and your thyroid hormone levels also decrease.

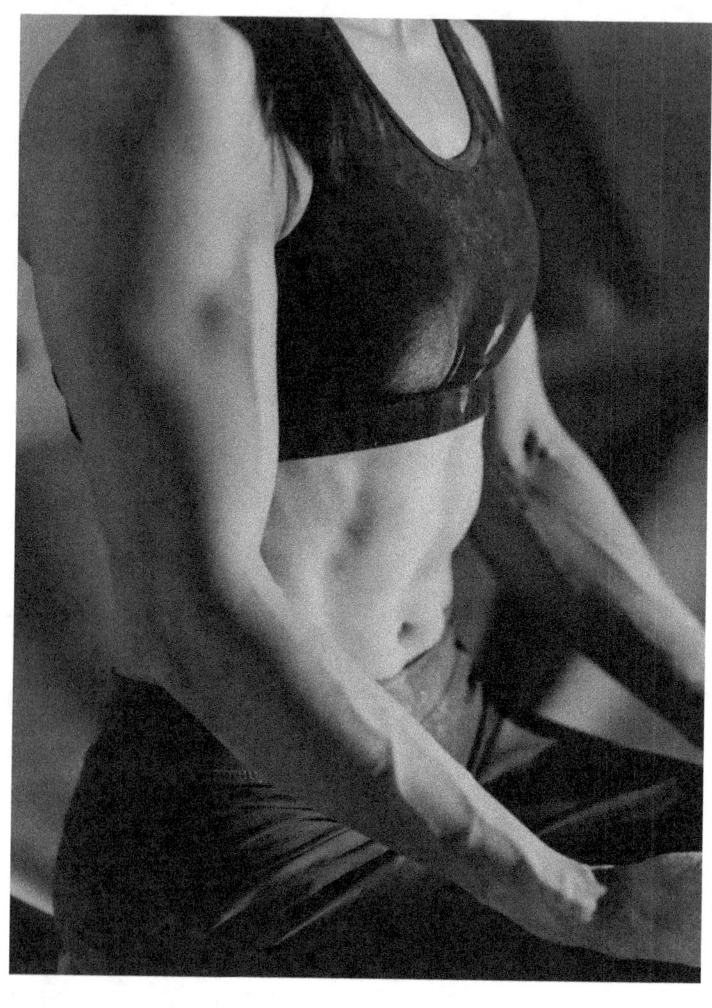

Cottonbro,pexels.com

The 50s:

This is the decade when your menstrual cycle stops, and you are officially menopausal when you haven't had your period in 12 consecutive months. Your androgen levels decrease. Your sleep is disrupted, which will definitely affect your performance in your exercise sessions. Hydrate sufficiently. The deficiency in your estrogen increases the risk of you getting osteoporosis. This is when you should increase your strength resistance training to maintain the integrity of the musculoskeletal system. Your walk becomes slower, and you are prone to knee injuries.

The 60s:

Many of the symptoms of menopause fade away, and you return to a stable and modulated body. By the age of 65, you are going to need to have your BMD checked out. If you come from a family that has a history of alcohol, smoking, or other related risk factors, then make sure you check your BMD before then. Your spinal column becomes curved and compressed. Make sure you spend enough time stretching, focus on decompressing your back and strengthen your back with exercise. Your feet flatten, which affects your gait and predisposes you to arthritis, bone spurs, bunions, calluses, lower back pain, hip pain, shin splints, and knee pain. Make sure your weight is on the lighter side so that you avoid a lot of pain. Increase your mobility exercises and lubricate your joints because they are much stiffer and less flexible. There is a prevalence of calcium deposition and osteoarthritis at this time. Your shoulder is most at risk of injury. Your fingers, hips, and knees lose cartilage. Your balance will also start becoming compromised. Train your proprioception.

The 70s, 80s, and beyond:

Your lean body mass continues to decline, and you experience a decrease of up to 30 % muscle mass loss. Your muscle fibers shrink, and your muscles become stiffer. Your heart rate decreases, and your heart becomes enlarged because there is an increase in blood pressure. Incorporate mild cardio in your exercise routine. Use Kegel exercises to strengthen your bladder because this is when you experience stress and urge incontinence. If your memory starts deteriorating, make sure you eat a diet high in vegetables and fruits. Your senses start losing their sensitivity. Your eyes become sensitive to glare, and your cataracts increase. Your hearing also declines. At this age, you bruise easily, and your skin loses elasticity which causes wrinkles. Stretch and get blood into your fascia, so your skin gets much-needed oxygen.

Chapter 4:

Training Psychology

"The most we can hope for is to create the best possible conditions for success, then let go of the outcome." Phil Jackson, author of *Eleven Rings*, wrote this. Phil is an absolute legend in basketball. He is probably the best basketball coach of all time. You can only let go of the outcome once you've produced the best possible conditions for success. This chapter is about just that; how to leverage your mind (first place to begin) so that it is conducive to empowering your performance in all aspects of your life. Whatever limits you place on yourselves are the limits that you will realize in your life. When you are confident in your ability to learn and to get better, you become an unstoppable force proving that strength is a movable object.

Skill Acquisition

	INCOMPETENT	COMPETENT
UNCONSCIOUS	Unconscious Incompetent	Unconscious Competent
CONSCIOUS	Conscious Incompetent	Conscious Competent

When you learn a new skill, you move from unconscious incompetent to conscious incompetent to conscious incompetent and finally conscious competent. Unconscious incompetent is when you know you don't know how to do the thing you want to learn, but you have no idea how much you don't know. Then you start learning the basics, and it sinks in that you don't know, and the path of competence opens into the horizon in front of you. You override your discouragement and tell yourself that this is a worthwhile skill to learn, so you put in the work and effort. Then you get better, and with enough time, you become proficient. Now you are consciously competent. When you work your way away from mere proficiency towards mastery, then the skill from the outside looks like it comes naturally to it. This is where you achieve what Mihaly Csikszentmihalyi called flow. "Flow is defined as an optimal state of consciousness, a state where you feel your best and perform your best. More specifically, the term refers to those moments of rapt attention and total absorption, when you get so focused on the task at hand that everything else disappears. Action and awareness merge. Your sense of self vanishes. Your sense of time distorts (either, typically, speeds up; or, occasionally, slows down). And throughout, all aspects of performance, both mental and physical, go through the roof." (Kotler, 2022)

Let's take my yoga journey. I started yoga because I wanted to increase my mobility. I was generally inflexible and knew that the older I got, the more likely I would end up injured. I wanted to be able to increase the suppleness of my muscles and improve my range of motion. So I downloaded beginner yoga classes and followed them. I've seen people in down-dog positions on TV, and it looked so easy until it was my turn to do it. My heels couldn't touch the floor, my upper arms were on fire, and I just couldn't maintain the position for too long until I retreated into a child's pose. That first yoga class was a complete eye-opener—I had no idea what I had gotten myself into. There were a lot of movements and a lot of technical alignment details, and there was also the big problem of regulating my breathing. When executing a difficult pose, I would hold my breath. This must be a common occurrence because the instructor kept reminding me to breathe. There were a lot of balls to juggle. Then as I progressed, I realized that yoga was about more than flexibility; there was strength, balance, cardio, and power, and did I mention breathing? Once I was able to see the bigger picture, then I was able to see how everything fits together.

The word yoga comes from Sanskrit, and it means to unite. And I finally cottoned on that flexibility was just one component that was being united with other components. I became consciously incompetent. I moved to the intermediate level, started practicing with different instructors, and even tried different yoga practices. I did ashtanga, hot yoga, power, and yin yoga, to name a few. Different instructors were able to show me my weaknesses very quickly. The biggest weakness was my core strength. My whole core was weak, so inversion poses (where the feet are in the air) took a lot of time to develop. As my core strengthened, I began to feel literally lighter and could control how my body moved better. Now I've moved on to the advanced level. While there are still some poses that I am working on, the ones that I learned in the beginning, I can execute in correct form without thinking about it. This process will be what it will be like for you in your exercising with weight journey.

Practice! Practice! Practice! Any motor skill that needs to be learned requires practice. But practice has a quality about it—it's not just quantity. It's easy, especially for our self-esteem, to practice the things we already know how to do, particularly as we age. But deliberate practice takes mere repetition to another level. "The hallmark of purposeful or deliberate practice is that you try to do something you cannot do—that takes you out of your comfort zone—and that you practice it over and over again, focusing on exactly how you are doing it, where you are falling short, and how you can get better." (Ericsson, 2016)

Mat Fraser, who has been crowned the fittest man on earth for a lustrum, says that weaknesses are opportunities waiting to be turned into strengths. Weaknesses point us in the direction we should be running towards. Practice can take place holistically and it can take place partially. In whole practice, the entire skill is focused on, and in part practice, the skill is broken down into its components. If a skill can be broken into independent parts, then part practice is the way to go. Whole practice is better applied with regards to skills whose parts are highly related and dependent on each other. If there is a high chance of injury, practice in parts. Tasks can be simplified, perhaps through the slowing down of a movement or using much lighter components. In yoga, there are straps and blocks that help in the learning of a new pose.

Depending on the skill, practice can be pure part practice where each movement is executed multiple times, then once each part has been grasped, it is all put together and executed consequently. Practice can also be progressive where you need to grasp a fundamental movement before adding to that movement. Variable practice includes practicing the different variations of the same skill. There are different types of squats: sumo, Bulgarian, landmine, overhead, goblet, Zercher, etc. These can improve your skill acquisition process.

This book leans heavily on the explicit instructional side so that you are equipped with the tools and guidance you need to be successful in your strength training journey. There are different instructional styles; the other two, apart from explicit, are guided discovery and discovery. Explicit instructions are the 'rules' for effectively performing a task; proprioceptive information, form, what the function of the exercise is, and direction of movement are examples of explicit instruction. In guided discovery, the overall movement goal is provided, but there are specifics that you will discover for yourself. For example, a yogi, while moving through different types of headstands, discovers that in the beginner headstands, the base is triangular to provide the greatest support. In discovery, you know what the goal is, but you have carte blanche on how you are going to get there. Picture the basketball player Robert Kurland as he dunks the ball into the basket. No one had ever dunked before, and it not only achieved the objective (get the ball in the net), but it didn't break any rules either. Pure discovery. Pure discovery requires time to play and tinker, but explicit instructions may also be limiting. Explicit instructions are also taxing attentionally. As I've mentioned at the beginning of this paragraph, this book makes use of a considerable amount of explicit instructions, and I don't think that is a bad thing when we are working with beginners. But I hope, as you proceed in your strength training journey and are comfortable with the fundamentals, you can start exploring and discovering things for yourself.

Feedback is paramount to progress in motor skill acquisition. There is the feedback that your own body will give you—this is intrinsic feedback. You lose balance, and you already know why that could have happened and adjust accordingly. Augmented feedback is provided by an observer or a wearable. They see something that you aren't aware of while you execute the task (knowledge of performance), or they are able to provide you information on whether you executed the task or not (knowledge of results).

Mind-Body Connection

I'm sure you've seen those guys in the gym flexing in between sets. They usually flex in front of a mirror. If you have seen this, and you have no idea what's happening: they are being mesmerized by their own pump. "The pump is when your muscles swell up during your workout, which is caused from the excessive amount of blood going into the muscle and filling it up the same way you would fill up a water balloon. Your muscles get a very full, tight feeling and your skin becomes tighter because of this." (NSCA, 2015). Beyond the pump, flexing between sets actually seems to work to improve strength. Contracting your muscles involves recruiting your upper motor neurons and lower motor neurons.

Dr. Andy Galpin, who has worked with a lot of athletes, says that awareness is important during workouts. In order to reap the largest benefits from a workout, your intentionality has to be turned on. If you take two people who are executing the same movement, one is just doing it because they want to get the exercise over and done with, and the other person is mentally prepared to make the most of the exercise. The one with intentionality reaps more benefits than the one who merely does the movement.

Proprioception, otherwise known as kinesthesia, is your body's ability to sense movement, action, and location. It's present in every muscle movement you have. Without proprioception, you wouldn't be able to move without thinking about your next step (Brennan, 2020). Tactile pressure assists in sharpening proprioception. When you are working out, and someone literally taps the muscle you are working on, that allows your mind to zero in on the muscle group and target it more. The same applies to a lifting belt that people use when they lift heavy weights. A lifting belt stabilizes the spine, but the fact that it's in contact with your body also reminds the lifter to keep their spine in the correct position by contracting their core. If a lifting belt is attached too tightly, then the lifter loses an opportunity to strengthen their core. But even in yoga, when the instructor lightly touches a part of your body, you are able to automatically align your body in the correct way. Touch is underutilized, primarily because of the times we live in where all touch can be misread as inappropriate. Please ensure that professionalism is maintained at all times.

There is an ideal performance state for athletes, but I think it applies to anyone who trains with the intention to make the most of their training. This state is characterized by an absence of fear, motor movements are automatic, attention is narrowly focused on the task at hand, there is a sense of effortlessness that comes from experience, there is a sense of personal control, and time and space distort where time seems to slow down (William & Krane, 1998). This sounds very similar to flow, which is exactly right. I would like you to become so in tune with your training program that every single exercise session yields benefits to you. In this peak state, there is no energy wasted.

Your ability to focus is tied to the idea of attention. "Attention is defined as the processing of both environmental and internal cues that come to awareness. A person's conscious attention is continuously bombarded with a variety of stimuli and internal thoughts to which it can be directed. The ability to inhibit awareness of some stimuli in order to process others is termed selective attention, and it suppresses task-irrelevant cues in order to process the task-relevant cues in the limited attentional space." (NSCA, 2015)

For you, cues could be your phone or the conversations of other people in the gym. Have a routine that you go through when your attention is disrupted. Something that helps you get back to the task at hand. To focus in general, I wear headphones in the gym and listen to music that has lyrics about excelling. Then if someone interrupts me during a workout, I take a few intentional breaths and am able to fully return to the exercise. Remember, your working memory has a limited capacity and can only deal with one thing at a time. So when intrusive thoughts enter, as the yogis say, "return to breath," and your instructor would say, "return to task." A few years ago, I was doing a deadlift, and a guy in the gym interrupted me and stood close by me. I felt rushed. I continued the lift, which was the worst thing I could have done at that point. I had lost focus, and instead of making sure my spine was neutral, I ended up in bed for a few days, not being able to sit up because my spine was wrecked. What I learned was that there would always be distractions, so whenever I get distracted during a lift, in particular, I take a step back, close my eyes and breathe. Then once I feel my annoyance has dissipated, I go back to the bar. There are always cues I go through (routine) before a deadlift. Feet are hip-width apart, symmetry in the position of my hands, back neutral, inhale and lift. If the lift is very heavy, I visualize a successful lift in my mind before I lift. Managing distractions and improving your selective attention is a skill that can be trained.

There are three progress steps that you go through when learning a new skill (Fitts & Posner, 1967). The first stage is the cognitive stage—when you think of every step in the exercise movement, which requires a lot of effort. The second stage is the associative stage, where you are more concerned with just doing the task instead of focusing on the details of the movement. In the third and final stage, you are able to automatically execute the skill, and you are relaxed. Automaticity and clarity will help you keep focus, which is what you must aim for.

There are two attentional styles that can be described in two domains: direction and width. The first domain describes whether your attention is introspective or extrospective; are you focused on how you are feeling or the environment. The second domain describes whether your frame is expansive or narrow. How these domains interact with each other is illustrated in the table below. Learn which frame you need to be in order to accomplish a certain part of the task (preparation, analysis, assessment, or action).

	External	**Internal**
Broad	Assess	Analyze
Narrow	Act	Prepare

Energy Management

A life of vitality is a life of energy management. Energy is not wasted on nonessentials like worry, anger, anxiety, or frustration. A life of vitality is a life of self-control. Emotions are basically the way that mental energy is accrued, maintained, depleted, and refreshed. They are temporary states that occur as a way for us to respond to things happening within and without us.

Emotions are both psychological and physiological, and they affect both physical and mental energy. They, therefore, can have adverse effects on how we perform or positive effects depending on how we interpret them. They are beneficial when they get us pumped, excited, motivated and make us feel good about ourselves. The effects of emotions can be averse when they are too positive (frenetic behavior) or too low (no arousal). We've seen people already lose the fight when they tell themselves how much they hate working out instead of getting excited about their exercise session. This is called the framing effect in psychology. "The framing effect can be described as a cognitive bias wherein an individual's choice from a set of options is influenced more by the presentation than the substance of the pertinent information. The salience of certain features over others, as well as the positive or negative connotations pertaining to the information, is more likely than the actual information itself to determine the recipient's response." (Perera, 2021). So when we don't have perspective when it comes to our emotions, they can affect how we show up to our training sessions and how hard we apply ourselves during them.

In the chapter on adaptations, I discussed how the body needs different stimuli or it plateau's. When you go to the gym and do the same thing daily, your body can anticipate that and stop making you stronger as a result. Even you get bored when your strength training is monotonous. The key term here is arousal. Arousal is how motivated a person is to do something at a particular time, and it involves both psychological and physiological activation. When you are fired up, you are ready to go, and you experience a large sense of control and focus. When you are emotionally flat, you are directionless and unmotivated to work out. When a performer does not experience any arousal, it usually means that they are not going to perform well at all. A little arousal is necessary. This arousal is sometimes called state anxiety and should not be confused with trait anxiety. State anxiety can be positive or negative, while trait anxiety is just bad because it's chronic and a personality disposition. Trait anxious people worry about things that are irrelevant to the task at hand. State anxious people can use their anxiety to tune in to the task more acutely. "State anxiety is the actual experience of apprehension and uncontrolled arousal. Trait anxiety is a personality characteristic, which represents a latent disposition to perceive situations as threatening." (NSCA, 2015)

A lot of women find training with weights threatening, and before, they are already preoccupied with failing or looking silly, so they shy away from the weights when the weights are their ticket to better health and resilient bodies. State anxiety is ineffective when you are tense, as your heart is racing and negative thoughts enter your mind. We usually feel like this when we are uncertain about an event (present or future). Before their first weight workout, women can experience this psychological inefficiency; they fear failing, their egos are involved, it feels like their self-esteem is at risk, and they think they are going to do much worse than they actually are. They start catastrophizing. Then when they get to the gym, they walk right by the weights. As this proceeds, I hope you become more and more comfortable with weights and how to handle them. I will be removing a lot of decision-making responsibilities to help you become more comfortable around weights with clear, simple, direct instructions.

When the word stress is mentioned, most of us go to the negative type. This is called distress, and we feel distressed. Maybe work or relationships aren't going well, and we experience negative stress. On the other side, a less utilized word is eustress which is positive stress. Sounds like an oxymoron, but it isn't. Stress is defined as an imbalance between physical or physiological demands and our capability to meet that demand. The consequences of failing to meet that demand are important to us. Distress leads to anxiety, and eustress leads to mental energy.

The less familiar you are with exercises, the more you want your arousal to be under control so that you can be calm enough to learn the technique and form. This stage is known as the stage of analysis, and it requires you to think about the steps of the movement. All you are thinking about attentionally is executing the move correctly, and we don't want you to be cognitively overloaded. As you proceed to acquire skills and become proficient in technique, then you are generally able to deal with less than optimal arousal states and still execute the exercise well. Simple, easy-to-execute tasks can handle a higher arousal state, but the more complexity is introduced in exercises, the arousal has to be kept low.

The Individual Zones of Optimal Functioning (IZOF) theory was developed by Yuri Hanin, and these are fancy words for saying that different people respond to different levels of arousal in different environments. For example, some of my clients who enjoy Zumba and like the fast pace, high-impact classes respond very differently when things slowdown in yoga. They will be aroused for both classes but will have different types and levels of arousing. Similarly, a spinning client might feel anxious when having to move to Zumba with all its directional changes, eccentric movements, and coordination. And not all positive arousal is good. Feeling too comfortable in a session can lead us to not perform as well.

In order for us to learn a new skill or effectively perform a motor skill, then we have to be motivated. "Motivation can be defined as the intensity and direction of effort." (NSCA, 2015). One of the taglines of fitness YouTubers, Buttery Bros is, "You've gotta want it!" and you really do gotta want it. There are two types of motivation: intrinsic and extrinsic motivation. Intrinsic motivation comes from an internal need to be competent and autonomous. People who are intrinsically motivated are driven by their love to participate in that activity, and the external rewards or punishments that come with that are but secondary. They derive deep enjoyment from the activity and want to learn and improve simply to get better. This type of motivation is maintained through gaining competence and the ability to exercise autonomy. When you set a performance or process goal and you achieve it then it becomes a positive feedback loop for you to continue. If you are going to train by yourself, then the self-autonomy can take care of itself, but if you are going to have a trainer, then ask your trainer to allow you to make certain decisions regarding your training program. The trainer would still be the authority, but if the entire training program is prescriptive, then interest and drive can wane. Extrinsic motivation is a motivation that comes from the outside environment: trophies, awards, praise, money, social approval, and a fear of punishment. People usually have both extrinsic and intrinsic motivation present, but you would want to lean towards the intrinsic for a longer arch of participation.

Achievement motivation "refers to a person's efforts to master a task, achieve excellence, overcome obstacles, and engage in competition or social comparison." (NSCA, 2015). When you take two athletes with the same skill level, the one who has a greater penchant for competition will be better. Society finds competition very tolerable and actually encourages it in sport—it's actually termed competitive sport. When competition leaves the field and courts and comes into other parts of life, then there is general disdain, especially among us women. An appetite for competition is not a bad thing. Don't get me wrong, it can really be taken to the extreme, but when applied correctly, it can elevate your performance demonstrably. In 2021, the movie *The Novice* came out, and it was about a young woman who joins the rowing team in college but goes to extreme lengths to outcompete everyone. She even put her life at risk by staying in the water while there was lightning. This young lady, unfortunately, has mental issues, and her level of competition has consumed everything else and become unhealthy. When competition becomes the main driver, then the likelihood of an injury or permanent damage increases. Remember, people who are intrinsically motivated, the "for the love of the game" people want to be able to continue playing for as long as they can, getting better and better with time.

They are not going to risk their lives and quality of life to win at all costs. But you and I are not athletes, so how do we show up to strength training sessions? The rule is simple: Outcompete yourself, be better than you were yesterday. Progress. The slightest change in adaptation will make you fitter.

Motive to Achieve Success (MAS) and the Motive to Avoid Failure (MAF) are the two conflicting personality traits that we human beings have. MAS refers to the capacity of being proud of your achievements, continually seeking to be challenged in your skills, and periodically evaluating your abilities (McClelland, 1953). The MAF personality trait is powered by a need to protect your ego and self-esteem. Remember, "your ego is not your amigo." It should always be put in check. We want to get stronger, and we must hit the golden mean between not doing enough (fear of failure) and doing too much (fear of losing face). Ryan Holiday says, "the obstacle is the way." Challenges are good for us, and we should neither avoid them nor be reckless in how we approach them. The path to strength will come with its own challenges, and we know that the MAS must override the MAF. There are no threats, just opportunities to improve our skills.

Positive reinforcements are the positive actions (object, praise, prize, rewards) that follow as a result of a certain behavior (operant) occurring. Negative reinforcements work in a similar way, except the actions that follow a failure to execute a certain behavior are negative, i.e., something gets taken away or something you do not want happening happens. Reinforcements focus on what you are doing correctly and therefore provide positive feedback. Therefore, you want to be focused on the task at hand. Reinforcements help improve people's self-esteem, self-efficacy, and confidence and produce long-term memories of success. Reinforcements work best with a coach or instructor, but I've personally used positive reinforcements when working out. When I actually get to the gym and complete a workout, I reward myself with a latte (no sugar, that would be undoing all the hard work I've put in). Even in the middle of a training session, if I execute an exercise in good form, I literally say, "Well done, Elrey, that was good form."

Psychological Techniques

"The greatest discovery of my generation is that human beings can alter their lives by altering their attitudes of mind." William James, who is considered the father of psychology, wrote this. All behavior is preceded by thoughts, beliefs, perceptions, and attitudes. In order for you to become stronger, you have to believe that you can become stronger. It's the Henry Ford quote, "Whether you believe you can or you can't, you are right." Our desired behavior is ultimately up to us. In order for us to be able to behave in desired ways, then we need to sharpen our mental skills. Like any other skills, they can be learned and optimized over time.

Diaphragmatic Breathing

"It turns out that when breathing at a normal rate, our lungs will absorb only about a quarter of the available oxygen in the air. The majority of that oxygen is exhaled back out. By taking longer breaths, we allow our lungs to soak up more in fewer breaths. The fix is easy: breathe less. But that's harder than it sounds. We've become conditioned to breathe too much, just as we've been conditioned to eat too much. However, with some effort and training, breathing less can become an unconscious habit."" (Nestor, 2020). How we breathe affects how we perform. As explained above by the breathing expert James Nestor, our performance is being lost to the environment due to our breathing inefficiencies. Diaphragmatic breathing allows us to decrease these inefficiencies but also helps us in managing our arousal. It precedes any other mental training techniques. Physiological effects of this type of breathing are experienced through the relaxation of muscle and alleviation of any tension, and your heart rate slows down and stabilizes. In diaphragmatic breathing, you draw your attention to your abdomen. People tense their shoulders when they breathe intentionally, so they should relax their shoulders. The abdomen should distend as you inhale—you would want to inhale to your maximum capacity. Air fills the lower abdomen, then moves to the mid-chest, then the upper chest, and exhales in the opposite direction. Everything in yoga is linked to the breath; in fact, you breathe into the spaces where you feel tightness, and when you exhale, the tissue is loosened. Breathing is indispensable to progress in yoga, but the same is true in every other sphere of life.

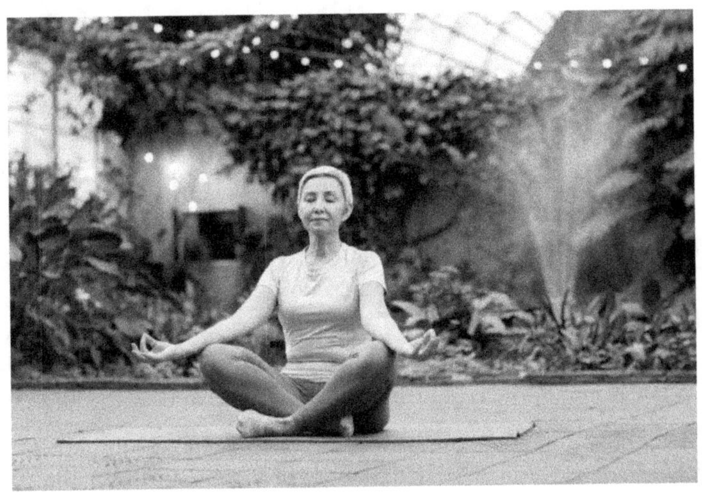

Marcus Aurelius, pexels.com

Nestor writes, "For every ten pounds of fat lost in our bodies, eight and a half pounds of it comes out through the lungs; most of it is carbon dioxide mixed with a bit of water vapor. The rest is sweated or urinated out. This is a fact that most doctors, nutritionists, and other medical professionals have historically gotten wrong. The lungs are the weight-regulating system of the body". Whether you are trying to lose weight or gain strength, it begins with your breath.

Self-Efficacy

Self-confidence improves performance, and the amount of confidence you have is a stronger predictor of performance than physiological arousal. Self-confidence is the general feeling that you can execute a behavior you want to execute. Self-efficacy is a proponent of self-confidence. Self-efficacy is a measure of your ability to execute a specific task. A highly self-efficacious person harbors no doubts regarding their ability to successfully execute a task, even if the person experiences some sort of failure. There are a number of sources that contribute to a person's self-efficacy: past accomplishments of success and failure, vicarious experiences gained through watching others perform the task, verbal persuasion from self and others, being able to use imagery, and seeing one execute the task, physiological states (highly efficacious people find physiological states facilitative and not debilitative) and emotional states (Bandura, 1977). When I do my warm-ups in my exercise session, I generally stream other people who are doing what I am about to do. It always makes me excited to watch someone do what I want to do. My self-confidence has not always been high, and I've been able to improve my self-confidence by improving my self-efficacy. One task at a time. I've been active most of my life, but I only started strength training a few years ago. I overcame my fear and asked the staff at the gym how machines that seemed tricky worked or watched other gym members or YouTubed (saving grace). But I was able to figure it out. I was surrounded by people who had figured it out, and that meant I, too, was able to figure it out.

Skill by itself will never get you to your A-game. You need to believe that you are capable of becoming strong. Your level of self-efficacy has a direct influence on how you make decisions. If you are highly self-efficacious and you believe you can become stronger, then eat food that will make you stronger. It's also important to remember that you can be high in self-efficacy even if you fail. This is when self-efficacy pulls us through. When we do something, and we fail at the task, those low in self-efficacy will accept the failure as proof that they should have even tried in the first place. On the other hand, someone high in self-efficacy will see failure as information and a challenge to be surmounted with just the right strategy or adjustment. "Self-efficacy influences people's choice of activity, their level of effort in that activity, and how much persistence they will have in the face of challenging obstacles." (NSCA, 2015)

Self-Talk

This section is a relevant segue from the previous section. You cannot be high in self-efficacy while your self-talk is negative. Your intrapersonal communication, as it's otherwise known, is the inner dialogue that you have with yourself. It is the things we utter out loud and in our heads as well. When we do something new or learn a new skill, it's that soundtrack playing in the background. The three categories of self-talk are positive, negative, or instructional. The different categories are described further in the following table.

SELF-TALK CATEGORIES			
	Positive	**Negative**	**Instructional**
Description	• Encouraging • Motivational • Reinforcing	• Anger • Discouragement • Doubt • Negative judgment	• Specific direction • Focus on necessary

			performance cues for a skill or strategy
Examples	• "Let's go!" • "I can do this!" • "I am ready!"	• "You suck!" • "You can't do this" • "What were you thinking?"	• "Keep your torso upright!" • "Feet shoulder-width apart!"

It has been found that performance improves due to positive and instructional self-talk in the lab, but outside of the lab, there are other factors that would need to be considered. Positive self-talk and instructional talk both are context-specific. Negative self-talk, however, is completely detrimental to performance because you end up focusing on irrelevant cues, can provoke negative emotions, and can then diminish confidence.

Goal Setting

"Goal setting can look different depending on an individual's lifestyle, values and definition of success. Your goals are unique to you and don't need to look like anyone else's. The classic goal-setting definition boils down to the process of identifying something you want to accomplish and establishing measurable objectives and timeframes to help you achieve it. Goal setting can help you in any area of your life, from achieving financial freedom to adopting a healthy diet. When you learn how to set goals in one area of your life, it becomes easier to set them in other areas. Setting progressive goals that allow small wins helps you move on to larger achievements. These small goals lead to progress, which is the only thing you really need to feel fulfilled and happy." (Robbins, 2022). Goal setting will increase your psychological development and how you execute tasks. Goal setting motivates you to prioritize efforts, increasing efforts because goal attainment is important, and you feel that you are making progress as you move towards your goals.

There are two types of goal setting: outcome-based and system or process-based goals. People like focusing on outcome goals as opposed to system goals which are more effective. System goals are all those goals that are within your purview. It is the daily habits that you build that will take care of the outcome. Effort yields results. So if you want to gain strength overall, you need to focus on the daily habits of showing up to training sessions, making sure you sleep at a certain time, progressing your weight, etc. All these things are in your control. Outcome goals, in contrast, we have little control over. And sometimes, they seem so far from us as to be perceived as unattainable. This can be discouraging. As James Clear of Atomic Habits says, "You do not rise to the level of your goals. You fall to the level of your systems."

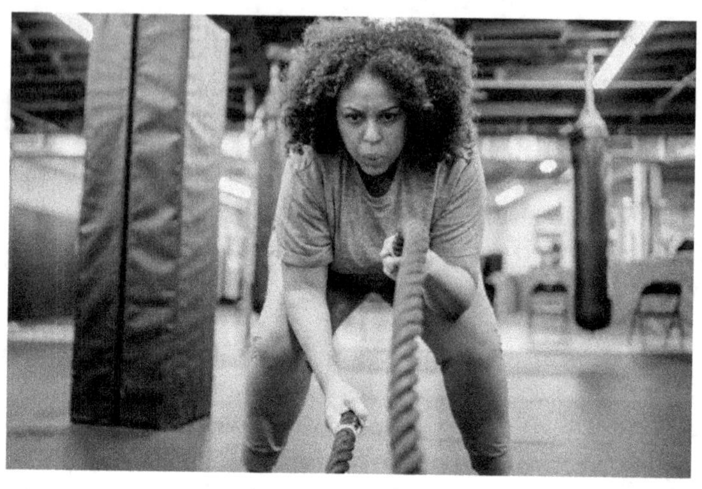

Julia Larson, pexels.com

Another goal categorization includes delineating between short-term and long-term goals. Short-term goals are the ones that are easier to achieve because they are not a far-fetched jump from where you are. They increase self-efficacy and confidence and your likelihood of success. You do not get bored either, as you would with a long-term goal that is not broken down into milestones. Our goal is to be strong throughout the rest of our lives, which can be a very long-term goal, so we need to break it down into short-term goals—this is how this book has been structured. Ultimately your short-term and long-term goals cannot be in conflict. They have to be aligned. The acronym SMARTER is the most widely used heuristic regarding goal setting. Goal setting has to snake use of Specific, Measurable, Actionable, Realistic, Timely, Enthusiasm, and Reviewed. People's goals are usually very vague. Even saying you want to become strong is a vague goal. But get excited about your goals. It's pretty exciting to get stronger, and that is how we should view our goals. It's not "I have to go to the gym, it's "I get to go to the gym." Lastly, review is a critical component of goal setting. Usually, when we start with a goal, there are a lot of things we are uncertain about, recall the quadrants we discussed in the previous chapter, and so we don't quite know the lay of the land per se. The process of reviewing is to assess our goals. Are the systems we have put in place working? Is there progress? Do we need to do something differently? Perhaps life gets in the way, and we aren't able to go to the gym in the afternoons anymore, etc. We constantly need to review the goals we've set and make sure that everything is conducive to our attainment of the goal. "Optimal goal setting requires knowledge of the exercise sciences in both biophysical and behavioral domains. The efficacy of goals for improving athletic performance lies in their relevance to the physical needs of the athlete." (NSCA, 2015)

Training Psychology Across the Decades

Training psychology links to the different psychology that women in their different decades experience. Motivation, self-talk, self-confidence, and goal setting in your general life will mostly correlate to all these aspects within the gym. And if you are battling on the confidence side, then picking up weights in the gym will do wonders for your confidence in the gym and the rest of your life.

The 20s:

You are most impatient and are quick to quit something if the results are slow. You experience a lot of self-doubt as well. When you start your strength training journey, do not give up when it seems as if it's not yielding any results. A lot of women in their 20s, because of the new workspace and living in new geographical locations, experience profound loneliness. They feel like they are becoming a different person and feel they are outgrowing their friends. They don't keep up with their old friends. As you begin your strength training journey, join a gym and make new friends. Don't see new situations as isolating but get a gym buddy who can help you stay motivated and see this through. You are very uncertain about a lot of things, including your career, relationships, and whether you are good enough or not. Make your strength training journey a staple, be consistent, and it will help tether you when the uncertainty climbs. You do a lot at work, and some of you are still studying as well, so time may be limited. Make your exercise sessions a big rock in your life. Social anxiety, lack of self-esteem, and shyness will all improve as you lean into strength.

The 30s:

This is when most people start having children and having families. The different changes your body will undergo coupled with the fact that you have different priorities now (you are more concerned with building a family) are where you are. Time becomes restricted in a different way than it was in your twenties. You are taking care of other people, and because of this, you may neglect yourself at this time. As rewarding as raising children is, make sure that you are pouring from a full cup. Fill your cup first so that you are not overwhelmed. Employ a lot of diaphragm breathing and mindfulness practice. Get strong in the gym, and you feel very empowered and more capable, and you will also be able to channel any feelings of frustration or stress that come with taking care of a family.

The 40s and 50s:

Abigail Stewart conducted a study to find out how middle-aged women's personalities change over time in four areas: identity, generativity, confident power, and concern about aging. "Identity is usually thought of as an accomplishment of adolescence... [it] was proposed that women might not develop identities in late adolescence and early adulthood as men did. Instead... women develop them later, in the context of intimate relationships." (Stewart, 2001). There is a positive correlation between women's well-being, self-esteem, and life satisfaction with identity development. Once their identity has consolidated, self-esteem soars, and they are highly motivated to do things that are good for them.

Women also experience a midlife generativity crisis as well as men, although it is hardly spoken of. This is the need to make a positive impact on and contribution to the next generation. "The crisis results in a capacity and commitment to care—for ideas, cultural products, institutions, values, and people." (Stewart, 2001). Since generativity is a long-term preoccupation and is only accomplished later in life, it affects the mental health of women in the later years.

Middle-aged women are known to be particularly productive, competent, and responsible. This is when women feel that they are in charge of themselves and their worlds. Confidence is very high, and women can generally cope with a lot more. Women in their middle ages are most likely to sign up for strength training. They are generally highly motivated, and their general competence would be a motivating factor for them to do well in their strength training regimen.

Mortality salience is "the awareness of the inevitability of one's own death, generates a state of anxiety that triggers a defense mechanism for the control of thinking that affects different human activities and psychological processes." (Gordillo, 2017). It's been assumed that women in their middle ages start experiencing anxiety about death, but that is not true. Women in their middle ages feel the most stable and satisfied about themselves and life. Mortality salience becomes a huge factor in the elderly. The only reason we don't see more middle-aged women in the gym is because society has relegated it as a young people's playground, but I am very sure that once that barrier is overcome, then middle-aged women will dominate and take to strength training with steely determination and fervor.

The following table itemizes the different feelings that women in their middle ages may feel (Stewart, 2001).

FEELINGS ABOUT LIFE SCALES

Identity Certainty
- a sense of being my own person
- excitement, turmoil, confusion about my impulses and potential
- coming near the end of one road and not yet finding another
- feeling my life is moving well
- searching for a sense of who I am
- wishing I had a wider scope to my life
- anxiety that I won't live up to opportunities
- feeling secure and committed

Generativity
- feeling needed by people
- efforts to ensure that younger people get their chance to develop
- influence in my community or area of interest
- aa new level of productivity or effectiveness
- appreciation and awareness of older people
- having a wider perspective
- interest in things beyond my family

Confident Power
- feeling powerful
- feeling more confident
- feeling that I have the authority to do what I want

- not holding back when I have something to offer
- having an accurate view of my powers and limitations
- feeling I understand how the world and other people work

Concern About Aging
- looking old
- thinking a lot about death
- knowing there are things I'll never do
- feeling less attractive than I used to be
- feeling men aren't interested in me

The 60s:

This is when mortality salience rears its head. We are winding down in our careers, and the children are growing up and leaving the nest. We have more time on our hands than we used to, and we have less responsibility. This is when we feel the decline of age. This is when we should strength train. We have more time on our hands and we can really spend more energy with our health as a priority and have not much else competing for our attention.

The 70s and 80s:

The decline in our physical capabilities is felt the most at this age. Even our relational dynamics change. We may have to be moved to retirement homes or assisted living. This time is a challenge mentally. We have to face that there are things that we can no longer do anymore. Our self-esteem takes a huge knock. We feel that we are an inconvenience to those around us. Our cognitive skills start to decline, and we may have dementia (more prevalent among women). We may feel isolated, which is far worse than the isolation in our twenties because then our bodies were an ally. Okay, so this is a very glib view of our latter years. All of these can be stalled, and you can live a life of vitality in these years. But you have to make health decisions early in your life that will set you up for later in your life. I have a saying, "Take care of your body now while you still can so that it can take care of you later when you are unable to." Train for strength and reverse your biological clock. Stay positive about your life. Savor each day.

Personality Over the Decades

For the longest time, it's been believed that personality is fixed. Brent Roberts, a psychologist, says (Whitcomb, 2020), "Personality is a developmental phenomenon. It's not just a static thing that you are stuck with and can't get over," In the short term, you won't be able to see the changes, but long term, you can see how different you are now compared to a decade ago. The Big Five personality traits are Openness to experience, Conscientiousness, Extroversion, Agreeableness, and Neuroticism (OCEAN). A study conducted in 2000 analyzed 52 longitudinal studies with participants ages ranging from childhood to 70's analyzed these personality traits over time. The maturity principle in psychology describes how people become more extroverted, emotionally stable, conscientious, and agreeable as they grow older. The changing circumstances—work, family, studying—start to require more from us. "Over time you are asked in many contexts across life to do things a bit differently. There's no manual for how to act, but there are very clear implicit norms for how we should behave in these situations." (Whitcomb, 2020)

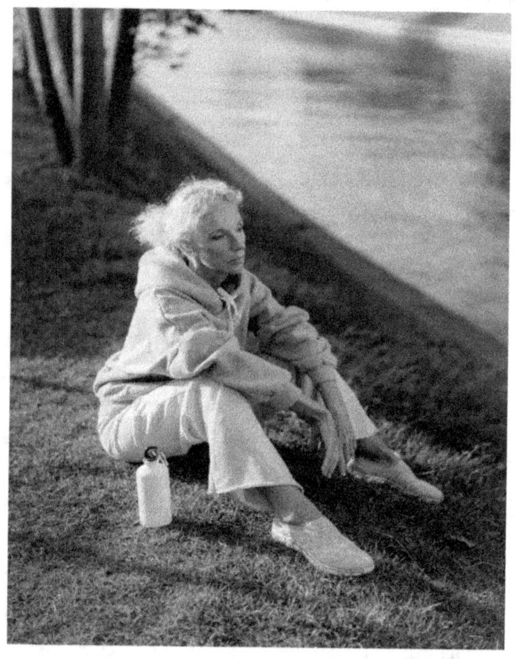

Cottonbro, pexels.com

Chapter 5:

Nutrition

As the aphorism goes, "you are what you eat." Good nutrition is the backbone for general health, development, growth, and tissue repair but also provides the fuel needed in order for you to be able to execute the movements in your training session. Nutrition plays a key role in preventing injuries and maximizing adaptations. Nutrition is not the easiest thing to navigate and figure out either, especially in this century where there are so many different diets and a lot of conflicting information regarding what to eat.

My Plate

The U.S. Department of Agriculture developed a food guidance system based on the 2010 Dietary Guidelines for Americans. It was developed to assist consumers in making better food choices. MyPlate consists of five food groups (fruits, grains, vegetables, protein, and dairy) that are based on a meal time visual. MyPlate provides calorific and portion guidance based on age and sex. There is also a dietary allowance for oils. MyPlate is a rudimentary tool to start with, particularly because it emphasizes that you eat a variety of food.

This is always a good sign because you will most likely get all the nutrients that you need. This section will be based on the assumption that no food groups have been left out. Vegans and any other food-excluding groups will not be catered for in this book. A diet across the different food groups will make sure that you meet your macronutrients (carbohydrates, protein, and fat) and micronutrients (vitamins and minerals).

Dietary Reference Intakes

People don't eat individual nutrients; they eat whole food, so any dietary recommendations must be in the form of food choices. MyPlate focuses on civilians who do not exercise. Dietary Reference Intakes (DRI's) are developed by the Food and Nutrition Board, National Academies, and the Institute of Medicine for people who are healthy. DRI's are a complete set of nutrient intakes and can be used when planning and evaluating diets for healthy people. They are composed of macros, micros, electrolytes, and water. They are centered on optimization and not just making sure that people aren't deficient. The DRIs consist of four things. The Recommended Dietary Allowance (RDA) is the average daily nutrient that will sufficiently meet the needs of most healthy people at each stage of life, taking sex into consideration. When an RDA can not be quantified, then Average Intake (AI) is used to guide average daily nutrient intake. The Tolerable Upper Intake Level (UL) is the maximum average daily nutrient that does not pose any health risks. The UL considers food, water, and supplements. The average daily nutrient intake is enough to meet the requirements of half the population at different stages of life and with different genders.

Most people are deficient in Vitamin E and magnesium. Foods rich in magnesium are nuts, seeds, and beans. Vitamin E is found in oils, nuts, and seeds. Potassium and fiber are low in people over the age of two. Another nutrient of concern beyond the ones already listed is calcium. Fortified beverages (milk, orange juice) and canned sardines are great sources of calcium, and fortified yogurt is a great source of vitamin D.

Macronutrients

A macronutrient is a nutrient that is required in large doses in the diet. There are three important categories of nutrients: protein, fat, and carbohydrates.

Protein

Every cell in the human body is made of proteins. When the body recovers after the breaking down of muscle to form new muscle, it's called protein synthesis. Protein that we consume is used to develop, grow, build and repair cells in the body; they also serve as enzymes, hormones, and transport carriers. Dietary protein is important to maintain health, cellular structure, and function. They are made of carbon, oxygen, hydrogen, and nitrogen. Any item that is preceded by the word 'amino' means that it contains nitrogen; therefore, amino acids are molecules that are most prevalent in nature. The human body consists of proteins made from about 20 individual amino acids. There are four that can be synthesized by the body, and these are called non-essential amino acids as they can easily be made by the body. There are nine amino acids that are essential, and they are provided for from outside the body, i.e., diet. The remaining eight amino acids are conditionally essential. In essence, when the body is healthy, it doesn't need amino acids but if the body is going through stress and illness, then it does. The quality of protein is determined by the content of amino acids and also the protein's digestibility. Protein digestibility is how much of the protein's nitrogen is absorbed during digestion and how able it is to provide amino acids that are imperative for growth. The different amino acids are summarized in the following table.

Essential	Nonessential	Conditionally Essential
Histidine	Alanine	Arginine
Isoleucine	Asparagine	Cysteine
Leucine	Aspartic acid	Glutamine
Lysine	Glutamic acid	Glycine

Methionine		Proline
Phenylalanine		Serine
Threonine		Tyrosine
Tryptophan		
Valine		

Proteins that are high in quality are highly digestible, and all the essential amino acids can be found in them. Proteins from animals (meat, fish, poultry, eggs, and dairy products) have all the amino acids. Soy is the only plant-based protein that has eight of the nine essential acids, but the drawback when it comes to plants is that they are less digestible than animal products. The digestibility can be improved through preparation and cooking. In general, foods have antinutritional factors, which are compounds that decrease the digestion and absorption of the nutrient, so less than what is available is used by the body. These antinutritional factors lead to a limit in the bioavailability of amino acids. The Maillard process is the process we use when we brown food while cooking. This browning of food is important because it increases the aroma and flavor of food, but it also increases the safety of food. Unfortunately, "the nutritive value of the food is moreover reduced by Maillard reactions, since amino acids (mainly the essential lysine) are destroyed, and/or cross-links between protein chains are formed, eventually leading to an overall reduction in protein solubility and digestibility." (Hurrell, 1990)

Since all plants are short of at least one essential acid, people who don't eat meat products, like vegetarians and vegans, would need to consume a variety of plant foods, including seeds, nuts, whole grains, vegetables, and legumes. Dietary recommendations specify protein but what they are actually recommending is amino acids. When cells break down and rebuild, this cell turnover requires amino acids. The recommendation for protein for adults (both men and women) above the age of 19, based on nitrogen balance studies, is 0.8 g of high-quality protein per kilogram body weight daily. Children, women who are pregnant or lactating, and teenagers need different dietary requirements. When you are exercising, and there is a caloric deficit in your body, you need even more protein. "Therefore, The Institute of Medicine (IOM) established an Acceptable Macronutrient Distribution Range (AMDR) for protein, which covers a wide range of protein intake. The AMDR is 5% to 20% of total calories for children ages 1 to 3 years, and 10% to 30% of total calories for children ages 4 to 18 years, and 10% to 35% of total calories for adults older than age 18 years. Men and women typically consume an average of 15% of their calories from protein." (NSCA, 2015).

The difference between the AMDR and DRI is that the DRI only takes in body weight while the AMDR takes low and high-calorie intakes into account. When it comes to people who exercise, the protein is the base, and all the other macros are added to meet the total calories needed. Most experts feel that we need much more protein than the RDA, especially since protein repairs tissue, management of weight, and bone health. High protein, low carbohydrate diets seem to be good for decreasing cardiovascular disease and metabolic syndrome, particularly in obese individuals. The more protein you eat, the quicker you reach satiety. The satiating effect of protein does depend on the form of the protein (liquid or solid), what time you ingest the protein, and also what other macros you are consuming at the same time. More calories are burned when the body digests protein more than any other macro because protein has the highest thermic effect on feeding. People who exercise need much more than the RDA of protein. People who train for endurance need 1.0 to 1.6 g of protein per kilogram body weight daily, and those who train for strength need between 1.4 to 1.7 g of protein per kilogram body weight daily. People who train a combination of both require between 1.4 to 1.7 g of protein per kilogram per body weight daily. Even if you are on a diet where your calories are reduced, your protein has to increase in order to preserve muscle tissue during weight loss. The best time to consume protein is just after exercise. The longer you wait, the more muscle sensitivity to amino acids decreases. The sooner you consume protein, the more acute the protein synthesis in the muscles. The accepted ratio of carbohydrates to protein is 4:1. Post-workout, eat about 20 to 48 g of protein. The older you are, the more you would eat on the higher grams side because sensitivity to amino acids decreases with age. The other macros are important as well, so you should not consume so much protein that there is no calorie room left for you. The following table lists the best sources of protein (Ronnberg, 2017).

BEST SOURCES OF PROTEIN
Feta cheese (10% fat)
Pork tenderloin
Turkey
Cottage cheese
Fat-free Greek yogurt
Chicken
Ground beef (5-10% fat)
Salmon
Mackerel
Mozzarella (20% fat)
Cheese (10% fat)
Sirloin
Shrimp
Tofu
Tuna

Cod
Game
Eggs

Carbohydrates

Carbohydrates are a source of energy. However, they are not an essential source because the body can break down amino acids and convert them into glucose. Carbohydrates are made of hydrogen, carbon, and oxygen, and they can be classified into three different types according to how many sugar units they have in them. Mono(one)saccharides, disaccharides, and poly(many)saccharides. The main monosaccharides are glucose, fructose, and galactose. The circulating sugar in the blood is glucose, and cells in the body live off glucose. The compound found in candy and sports drinks is glucose. Fructose has a sweeter taste than glucose. It is found in fruits and vegetables and in honey. One of the good things about fructose is that it causes less insulin release in the body compared to other sugars. Galactose is a combination of glucose and lactose. Disaccharides consist of sucrose, lactose, and maltose. The most common disaccharide is table sugar. It does occur in most fruits. Only mammalian milk has lactose. Maltose is the main carbohydrate in beer. While the other two are simple carbohydrates, polysaccharides are complex carbohydrates. Starch is a polysaccharide and is found in legumes, grains, and vegetables. Fibers are also carbohydrates, and they are characterized by being partially resistant to the digestive enzymes of human beings. The effects that fibers have on the body, depending on the type of fiber, include making you feel satiated for a longer period of time. Other fibers can increase water content, decreasing constipation and decrease how much cholesterol is absorbed into the blood. Other fibers stimulate a healthy microbiome (gut bacteria). Whole-grain food, vegetables, fruits, beans, peas, and bran are some sources of fiber. The DRI for fiber ranges from 21 to 28 g per day for women and 30 to 38 g per day for men. Glycogen is found in the body, with most of it being stored in the skeletal muscle and the remaining quantities being found in the liver.

The glycemic index is a ranking of carbohydrates in accordance with their digestion and absorption rate. Foods that are slow in being digested and absorbed are called low-GI foods, and they result in a rise in sugar levels much less than high-GI foods, and less insulin is released into the body. Insulin helps to decrease glucose in the blood by transporting it into cells. Low-GI foods have been connected to a decrease in obesity and other diseases. GI numbers are not consistent, however, and they are subject to variations in the ripeness of food, food processing methods, cooking and storage, and what they are consumed with. Beans, legumes, and whole grains are examples of low-GI foods. People who exercise can eat low-GI food and then replenish energy stores by consuming high-GI food after a workout. The glycemic load (GL) is the quantity of carbohydrates in a portion of food. Older adults should eat a low-GI diet because it improves insulin sensitivity and has fewer inflammatory markers. Chronic inflammation may lead to chronic diseases. Low-GI food decreases cardiovascular risk factors.

Carbohydrates can increase the time before you become exhausted in an endurance workout and can increase your work output in anaerobic workouts. Having enough carbohydrates allows the body to use the carbohydrates as fuel and spare protein. "Carbohydrate recommendations are largely based on the type of training. Aerobic endurance training 90 minutes or more per day at moderate intensity (70-80% VO2 max) should aim for 8 to 10 g of carbohydrate per kilogram body weight per day. [People] who benefit from this level of carbohydrate intake include those engaged in continuous aerobic activity such as distance runners, road cyclists, triathletes, and cross country skiers." (NSCA, 2015). People who train strength or sprint need around five to six grams of carbohydrates per kilogram of body weight daily. If you don't work out every day, then you can replenish your stores over the course of 24 hours. Remember that fat can be used as fuel as well, so if that is what you are going for (weight loss), then you wouldn't need to replenish stores fully. I recommend the following carbohydrates.

BEST SOURCES OF CARBOHYDRATES
Buckwheat
Beans/legumes
Whole grain bread
Rolled oats
Potatoes

Quinoa
Root vegetables
Brown rice
Sweet potatoes
BEST FRUITS/BERRIES
Oranges
Bananas
Blueberries
Grapefruit
Raspberries
Strawberries
Kiwi fruit
Plums
Pears
Apples
BEST SOURCES OF VEGETABLES
Eggplant
Avocadoes
Cruciferous vegetables (broccoli, cauliflower, cabbage,

kale)
Bell peppers
Lettuce
Asparagus
Spinach
Mushrooms
Tomatoes
Zucchini

The word lipid is a general category that contains fats and oils. The only lipid we are going to focus on is triglycerides because they are the ones that are found in most food and in the body. Fat is also made of hydrogen, carbon, and oxygen. Fats provide more energy than the other macronutrients because they have more hydrogen and carbon. Carbohydrates and proteins provide 4 kcal/g. and fats provide 9 kcal/g. There are different types of fatty acids that make fats. Saturated fatty acids are nonessential fats because the body can produce them, but because of how they are structured, they are less reactive. Unsaturated fatty acids are more reactive and can monounsaturated or polyunsaturated. Omega-3 and omega-6 fatty acids are the two essential polyunsaturated fats that are necessary for the development of healthy cell membranes, the brain, the nervous system, and the production of hormones. Omega-6 can be found in corn, soy, and safflower oil.

Unlike Omega 6, which is readily available, omega-3 is hard to come by. Food that contains omega-3 is fatty fish such as herring, trout, mackerel, halibut, and salmon. Omega-3 plays a role in decreasing blood pressure and antiarrhythmic effects in older adults. Foods such as canola oil, soy, walnuts, and flaxseed contain omega-3, but it has to be converted in the body for it to offer the above benefits. The aroma, flavor, and texture of food are owed to fat. All fats and oils have all three fatty acids, but there is one that is more predominant. Oils that are high in polyunsaturated fatty acids are oils from corn, soy, safflower, and sunflower. Peanut, olive, and canola oils are high in monounsaturated fatty acids, and saturated fatty acids can be found in most animal fats and tropical oils (palm and coconut). The adipose tissue, which is how fats are stored in the body, protects and insulates the organs, transports fat-soluble vitamins (A, D, E, and K), and regulates hormones.

Cholesterol is a form of fat that has a waxy sort of feel to it that is important in healthy cell function. It is used in the production of sex hormones, cortisol, vitamin D, and sex hormones. High levels of cholesterol, however, can cause a plaque build-up on artery walls called atherosclerosis. Blood is not able to pass through, which is why you could end up with heart disease or a stroke. Blood fats will increase when you eat a lot of refined carbohydrates, drink a lot of alcohol, gain considerable weight, and do not consume enough good fats. "The Scientific Report of the 2015 Dietary Guidelines Advisory Committee recommends avoiding partially hydrogenated oils containing trans fat and limiting saturated fat to less than 10% of total calories and replacing saturated fat with unsaturated fat, particularly polyunsaturated fat. In addition, it is advised that sugars consumed be a maximum of 10% of total calories." (NSCA, 2015)

Fatty acids circulating in the blood and those that in the muscles are potential energy sources during exercise. The body has limited storage space for carbohydrates, but fat stores are large and can provide large amounts of fuel for exercise. When you are at rest or engaging in low-intensity activities, then the body uses fats as fuel, but as you increase your intensity, then the body prefers to burn carbohydrates instead of fats. The following table lists the fats you should be eating (Ronnberg, 2017).

BEST FATS
100% raw chocolate
Avocado
Chia seeds
Fatty fish
Fish oil
Seeds
Cocoa (preferably raw)
Coconut oil
Flaxseed oil

Nut butter
Olives
Cold-pressed canola oil
Grated coconut
Butter

Micronutrients

Vitamins are organic compounds that are needed in very small quantities in the body, but that also carry out specific metabolic functions. They facilitate certain reactions in the body. The following table describes food sources of vitamins and what the vitamin does in the body. There are water-soluble vitamins, such as all the B vitamins and vitamin C, which dissolve in water and are carried by the blood. The body extracts what it needs from these vitamins and then flushes out what's left; therefore, taking more of these vitamins will not do anything except increase the amount of waste product that you urinate. Then there are fat-soluble vitamins (A, D, E, and K) which are transported by the fat in the blood and stored in the body's fat tissue. These are not to be consumed in excess. Dizziness, liver damage, nausea, headaches, and joint pain are some of the side effects of having too much vitamin A in the body. It can be fatal, and you should look out for it in supplements particularly. Vitamin D can increase blood calcium which can lead to the calcification of tissue as well as arrhythmias and kidney and heart damage. Vitamin E thins the blood, and an excess can increase the likelihood of a hemorrhagic stroke.

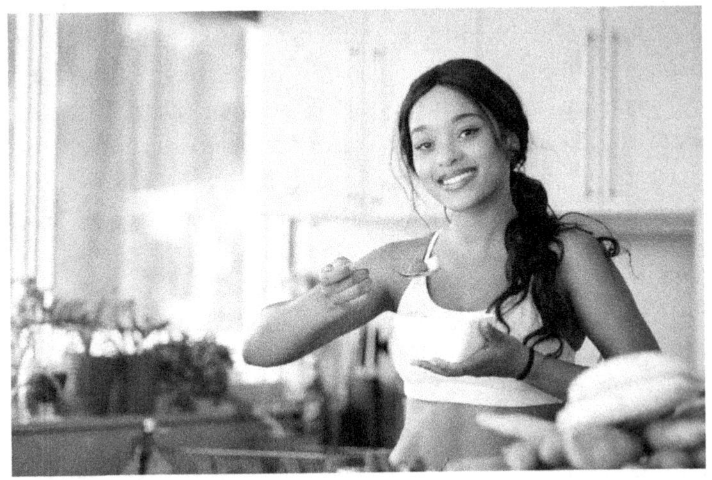

Nathan Cowley, pexels.com

Calcium and Iron

Minerals give the structure of bone, nails, and teeth, and they also perform a lot of different metabolic functions. Calcium, for example, is important for bone and tooth formation, muscle contraction, and nerve transmission. Iron transports oxygen and is necessary for the metabolism of energy. The major minerals consist of iron, magnesium, calcium, phosphorus, and electrolytes (potassium, chloride, sodium). Minerals maintain electrolyte balance in the body and bone health. When you don't consume enough iron, then you can develop anemia, and in the case of calcium, insufficient amounts can lead to low BMD, which poses a future health risk for further developing osteopenia or osteoporosis. The most prevalent deficiency in the world is iron deficiency. It appears in three stages: depletion, marginal iron deficiency, and anemia. "The National Nutrition and Health Examination Survey (NHANES) found that approximately 16% of teenage girls aged between 16 to 19 and 12% of women aged 20 to 49 were deficient in iron. In some studies, examining iron deficiency in female aerobic endurance athletes, more than one in four women tested positive for iron deficiency." (NSCA, 2015).

Some of the symptoms of iron deficiency include fatigue, weakness, headaches, poor concentration, hair loss, decreased exercise capacity, dry mouth, shortness of breath, and pica. Pica is an eating disorder where people eat non-food items such as ice, sand, coal, etc. Postmenarchal women, pregnant women, infants, and toddlers have the highest rates of deficiency mainly because they need iron the most. There are two types of iron found in food: heme iron and nonheme iron. Heme is better because it is easily digested and absorbed into the body. Foods that have heme iron are poultry, red meats, and fish. Cereals, grains, and vegetables provide nonheme iron. With regards to calcium, when it is insufficient, then it is drawn from the bone. It is important for the attainment of peak bone mass, as it keeps teeth strong and assists the functioning of nerves, blood vessel expansion, contraction, and enzyme and hormone secretion.

The following table lists the best seasonings to add to your food (Ronnberg, 2017).

BEST SEASONINGS

Balsamic vinegar
Lemon and lime juices
Curry, red and green
Cinnamon
Cardamom
Coconut milk
Crushed tomatoes
Marinated garlic cloves
Gingerbread spices
Pesto
Salsa
Tabasco hot sauce
Garlic
Apple sauce

Fluid and Electrolytes

Forty-five to seventy-five percent of your body is made of water. Water functions as a shock absorber, lubricant, building material, solvent, body temperature regulation, nutrient carrier, and waste product remover, and it maintains blood pressure. When you exercise, you lose water in sweat, and if you don't drink enough fluids, then you can end up in a hypohydrated state. Your core temperature increases, the volume of blood plasma decreases, and there is an increased heart rate. You will get tired much quicker in this state. Older people are more likely to become dehydrated because less fluids are consumed as people become older. It is recommended that men and women drink 3.7 l and 2.7 l per day, respectively. Even diuretics (coffee and tea) are sources of fluid. People with larger bodies are most likely to become dehydrated. You don't want to lose more than 2% of your body weight in sweat during exercise. A heuristic for determining your hydration status is to measure yourself before and after a workout in minimal clothing.

Electrolytes make sure that the water you consume is used efficiently by the body. Without electrolytes, water just travels through the body, and you urinate it. Sodium keeps water in the body. When you sweat, you lose electrolytes which are important for muscle contraction and nerve conduction. People sweat differently, some profusely and others mildly, with the same amount of work. If you are a sweater, add salt to your food and electrolytes to your drinks. Salt has been vilified a lot in society, but it is so important for the effective functioning of the body. When you don't take in enough salt, you risk hyponatremia, which results in swelling, headaches, nausea, muscle cramps, disorientation, and lethargy. This usually happens when people drink too much water. Sports drinks do not provide all the necessary electrolytes in the quantities you need; therefore, you have to eat food that supplements these. Always start your workout in a hydrated state. If you drink fluid during your workout, make it a high in carbohydrates drink. Drink post-exercise to replenish lost fluids.

Overweight and Obesity

People are considered overweight if their Body Mass Index (BMI) is between 25 and 29.9, and they are obese if their BMI is 30 or greater. BMI is calculated as a quotient of your mass and the square of your height in kg and m, respectively. These conditions increase a person's risk of dying from hypertension, heart disease, type 2 diabetes, sleep apnea, cancer, osteoarthritis, and dyslipidemia. In the United States, obesity is considered a disease, and it affects 34.9% of adults and 17% of children. While the causes of obesity are extensive and involve genetic, environmental, social, cultural, behavioral, and physiological factors, obesity can be treated. Treatments range from pharmacotherapy, surgery, dietary therapy, physical activity, and behavioral therapy. If you are overweight, then your treatment should result in 10% weight loss within six months in order for it to be seen as an effective treatment. "Body

Mass Index should not be used as a diagnostic tool but instead as an initial screening tool to identify potential weight issues in individuals and to track population-based rates of overweight and obesity." (NSCA, 2015). Waist circumference is another way to assess disease risk with women having a waist circumference bigger than 35 inches (88 cm). Weight loss is a very intense process and will require tremendous dedication from you. Make sure that apart from a personal trainer, you have a mental health specialist who will help you navigate that process.

Sometimes there is a temptation for people to go to the extremes and experience rapid weight loss because they want to get to an ideal goal weight, usually for an event. Voluntary dehydration (diuretics, water and salt diets, sauna, wearing too much clothing in hot weather), fasting, laxative abuse, induced vomiting, and inappropriate use of thermogenic technologies are some of the ways this rapid weight loss can be achieved. This is very dangerous and can result in the loss of lean body mass, mood swings, fatigue, and headaches. Your performance and training will also be put in jeopardy. Other side effects of rapid weight loss include heat illness, dehydration, dizziness, muscle cramping, hormonal imbalances, hyperthermia, low blood pressure, suppressed immune system functioning, kidney failure, passing out, and death. If you have a history of any sort of eating disorder or unhealthy weight loss/gain manipulation, then please consult your doctor before proceeding with a strength training regimen. Weight loss has to be gradual and sustainable.

We are all familiar with anorexia nervosa, bulimia nervosa, binge eating disorder, and pica (I've mentioned it earlier in the chapter), but there is also another eating disorder called rumination disorder, where the person who has this disorder chews, swallows, and regurgitates food. ARFID stands for Avoidant/restrictive food intake disorder and is basically a disinterest in food because the consequences of eating are seen in a negative way. People who suffer from this disorder are malnourished.

The symptoms of anorexia nervosa are "thinning of bones, brittle hair and nails, dry and yellowish skin, growth of fine hair all over the body, mild anemia and muscle wasting and weakness, severe constipation, low blood pressure, slowed breathing and pulse, damage to the structure and function of the heart, brain damage, multiorgan failure, drop in internal body temperature, lethargy and infertility." (NCSA, 2015)

The symptoms of bulimia nervosa are "chronically inflamed and sore throat, swollen salivary glands in the neck and jaw area, worn tooth enamel, acid reflux disorder and other gastrointestinal problems, internal distress and irritation from laxative abuse, severe dehydration from purging of fluids and electrolyte imbalance which can lead to a heart attack." (NCSA, 2015)

All eating disorders can only be diagnosed and treated by a qualified health care practitioner.

Nutrition Across the Decades

The following table summarizes all the food that you should be eating in each decade, depending on the demands of life and your body (Brown, 2021).

THE BEST FOODS TO EAT IN EVERY DECADE			
20s	**30s**	**40s**	**50s**
Protein	Bone Broth	Fermented Foods	Eggs
Complex Carbohydrates	Super Foods	Natural Phytoestrogens	Basil
Nuts and Seeds	Bok Choy	Bright Veggies	Brazil Nuts
Hormone Balancing Food	Antioxidants	Heart Healthy Foods	High Fiber Veggies
Liver Cleansers	Fish and Eggs	Whole Grains	Turmeric
Iron	Folic Acid	Omega-3	Zinc
	Low-fat Dairy	Artichokes	Plant-Based Protein
	Rainbow of Veggies	Seaweed and Sunflower Seeds	B Vitamins
	Vitamin E	Coconut	

60s	70s	80s
Bright Veggies	Colorful Veggies	Bright Veggies
Fruits	Legumes	Whole Grains
Whole Grains	Fruit	Vitamin D
Fish	Whole Grain	Calcium
Beans	Fish	Low-fat Milk
Lean Meat	Eggs	Cheese
	Milk	Seafood
	Yogurt	Eggs
	Nuts and Seeds	Beans
		Nuts & Seeds

The following table is the estimated calorie needs of female athletes by activity level. Light activity level: walking, house cleaning, golf, sailing, working in a restaurant.

Moderate activity level: cycling, tennis, dancing, jogging.

Heavy activity level: basketball, climbing, soccer, running.

<table>
<tr><th colspan="3">ESTIMATED DAILY CALORIE INTAKE FOR WOMEN</th></tr>
<tr><td></td><td>kcal/lb</td><td>kcal/kg</td></tr>
<tr><td>Light activity level</td><td>16</td><td>35</td></tr>
<tr><td>Moderate activity level</td><td>17</td><td>37</td></tr>
<tr><td>Heavy activity level</td><td>20</td><td>44</td></tr>
</table>

Chapter 6:

Periodization

Tom Bilyeu of Impact Theory says, "Human beings are adaptation machines." He says we have an unparalleled ability to adapt to any changes. We resist change in general, but once we've accepted the change, then we easily adapt to it. This is not just limited to the ability to adapt behaviorally, to new situations or otherwise, but to the ability for our bodies to adapt to stimuli. This happens in exercise as well. If we do the same thing, day in and day out or week in and out, then our body adapts to this, and soon we aren't making any more progress. This is sometimes referred to as reaching a plateau. To prevent plateaus and ensure that you still make progress across the decades, then you need to periodize. "Periodization is the process of dividing an annual training plan into specific time blocks, where each block has a particular goal and provides your body with different types of stress. This allows you to create some hard training periods and some easier periods to facilitate recovery. Periodization also helps you develop different physiological abilities during various phases of training." (Holmes, 2022)

When your body experiences a new, novel, or higher stress than it previously experienced, then the first reaction of the body is a combination of fatigue, stiffness, soreness, and a depletion of energy stores.

This is dependent on the magnitude of the stressor. The body's reaction may last hours or even weeks. Then the body heads into the resistance phase, where it adapts to the stress and then returns to base functional capacity. The body can result in specific structural, mechanical, and biochemical adaptations if the stress is appropriately structured. This can lead to supercompensation. If the stressor is applied for a very long time, then your body moves into the phase of exhaustion. This is not what you want because it can take a long time to recover from, and your performance ability will be compromised. There are three things to look out for when you exercise to ensure that you don't wind up in the exhaustion phase: overtraining, monotony, and too much variety. Other factors that do not directly have anything to do with exercise are sleep, diet, interpersonal relationships, or work issues; these contribute to exhaustion as well.

Your body experiences fatigue, and if you allow enough time between stimuli, your fatigue lowers, and your body adapts. If you wait too long between stimuli, your body enters a detraining phase, and it's as if you never applied the initial stressor in the first place. You can still exercise while your body is not fully recovered and there is minor fatigue, but in those sessions, you would be using lighter weights, for example. Or you may work out different muscle groups the next day.

Periodization Cycles

The different periodization cycles are summarized in the following table. (NCSA, 2021)

PERIODIZATION CYCLES		
Period	**Duration**	**Description**
Multi-year plan	2-4 years	A four-year exercise plan is termed a quadrennial plan.
Annual training plan	1 year	The overall training plan can contain single or multiple macrocycles. It is subdivided into various periods of training, including preparatory, competitive, and transition periods.
Macrocycle	Several months to a year	This is an annual plan.
Mesocycle	2-6 weeks	Medium-sized training cycle, sometimes referred to as a block of training. The most common duration is four weeks. It consists of microcycles that are linked together.
Microcycle	Several days to 2 weeks	Small-sized training cycle; can range from several days to two weeks in duration; the most common duration is seven days. Composed of multiple workouts.
Training day	1 day	One training day that can include multiple training

		sessions is designed in the context of the particular microcycle it is in.
Training session	Several hours	Generally consists of several hours of training. If the workout includes > 30 minutes of rest between bouts of exercise, it would comprise multiple sessions.

Periodization Models

There are two types of periodization models: linear and non-linear periodization models. This may be a bit ironic since periodization is about moving linearity from exercise. Regardless, it was named linear periodization because the mesocycles are increased gradually through the increase of intensity over time. The non-linear periodization model is better described as the daily undulating periodization model because it involves large daily undulations in the load and volume of the selected core exercises. In the linear periodization model, the training load and volume are the same in that microcycle. The undulating model may cause greater peripheral fatigue and may increase the risk of injury and decrease your potential preparedness.

Overtraining

When you exercise, you do so in order to get stronger. You have to overload your body so that the adaptations can take place. It's a sweet spot, however, between overload and excessive overload. Overtraining takes place when the combination of training frequency, intensity, and volume is more than the body can take. This happens when there is also insufficient nutrient intake, lack of rest, or recovery. This can result in fatigue that starts affecting performance and can lead to injury. Maladaptation is the opposite of adaptation, and it's when you start moving the other way in gains. The recovery from overtraining can take weeks or months. There is a training strategy called Functional Overreaching (FOR), where you overtrain intentionally to build up the body's tolerance. Recovery for this takes a few days, and when it is applied well, overreaching can really improve your strength. Mismanaged, you can lose a lot of the hard work you would have put in to get stronger. When you overreach beyond your limits, it's called Non-Functional Overreaching. The body does let you know, however, that you are entering dangerous exercise territory. Your hormones get off-balance, your performance will decrease, you will get more fatigued, and even your vigor in your workouts will taper. "Heavy resistance training is accompanied by decreased vigor, motivation, and confidence; raised levels of tension, depression, anger, fatigue, confusion, anxiety, and irritability, and impaired concentration." (NSCA, 2015)

Periodization Across the Decades

Periodization in resistance training, in general, will target different adaptations that are all strength related.

Below is a model that you can use when you periodize for different strength types.

Phase	Hypertrophy/ Strength Endurance	Basic Strength	Strength / Power	Peaking
Intensity	Low to moderate 50-75% 1RM	High 80-90% 1RM	Low to very high 30-85% 1RM	Very high to very low 50% to 93% 1RM
Volume	High 3-6 sets 8-20 reps	Moderate to high 2-6 sets 2-6 reps	Low 2-5 sets 2-5 reps	Very low 1-3 sets 1-3 reps

Maintenance	Active Rest
Moderate to high 85-93% 1RM	Recreational activities (may not involve resistance training)
Low to moderate 2-5 sets 3-6 reps	

Chapter 7:

Resistance Training

"There are several things that can positively affect the adult skeleton, and most are a result of muscle use. When the body is subjected to heavy loads (job tasks or resistance training), the bone will increase in density and bone mineral content. If the body performs more explosive movements with impact, similar changes can occur. Some of the higher bone densities have been seen in people who engage in gymnastics or other activities that involve high-strength and high-power movements, some with hard landings. Other factors that influence bone adaptations are whether the axial skeleton is loaded and how often this loading occurs (frequency). Since the adaptation period of bone is longer than that of skeletal muscle, it is important to vary the stimulus in terms of frequency, intensity, and type." (NCSA, 2015)

Weight-Stack Machines vs. Free Weights

When it comes to resistance training, you can use (not limited to) free weights or weight stack machines that you see in the gym. Weight-stack machines provide better control of the direction and movement pattern of the resistance. Safety is a big advantage of weight-stack machines because the likelihood of tripping over a weight is reduced and for the weight to fall on you is low. From a technical point, very little skill is needed to make sure that the resistance is controlled. Weight-stack machines are designed in such a way that they can target specific muscles and muscles which would be difficult to access with free weights. Beginners are always encouraged to use machines because they are easier to use. Not much skill is required, and changing the weight is hassle-free. You don't have to literally pick weights up; you just move a pin up and down the different weights on the machine.

On the other hand, free weights offer whole-body training. Because most free weights are used while standing, more muscles are used in general. Free weights are good for bone mineralization, which is critical in the prevention of osteoporosis in the latter years of life. Keeping the weights stabilized requires the use of muscles, whereas machines take over that work for you. Free weights are more realistic in that picking up something heavy in real life and picking up heavy weights will require the same technique and strength. Machines are good at isolating a muscle group, while free weights are good at coordinating.

Friction

When one object tries to move against another object, a force develops that is trying to impede the movement. More strength is needed to start moving the object than to keep moving it once movement has been initiated. A sled is a perfect example of this. The more weights you put on it, the higher frictional resistance you have to overcome. This means you will need to put in more work.

Fluid Resistance

Fluid resistance is the resistive force that an object encounters when it is moving through a fluid. Remember, air is also a fluid, so throwing an object across a field involves fluid resistance. Sports such as swimming, golf, and rowing have to contend with fluid resistance. In 2021, a documentary was released where the greatest long-distance runner of all time, Eluid Kipchoge, broke a world record. He had assistance from other runners who ran alongside him in a formation that mitigated the effects of fluid resistance so that the fluid resistance wouldn't slow him down. Similarly, in cycling, the cyclists in the front are protecting the lead, but they, in turn, are getting a fluid resistance thrashing.

Even machines in the gym use hydraulics (water) and pneumatics (air), such as the rower and assault bike, respectively. These do not make use of any eccentric movements, so they would not be great to use in training for eccentric sports such as running.

Elasticity

Home use equipment mostly makes use of some sort of elastic component. Belts, bands, or springs offer resistance. The more the device is stretched, the higher the resistance provided. There is very little range of resistance provided by one belt, and therefore, its ability to make you stronger is limited, particularly when the principle of progressive overload needs to be applied. Resistance bands are great in the early stages of a training program, but there will come a time when your muscles need stronger stimuli.

Resistance Training Risks

All exercises carry a potential risk with them. Some exercises carry more than others. Resistance training has amongst the lowest rates of injury and is rated the same as walking. The higher injury rates come as a result of running or aerobics (NSCA, 2015). Even though injury through resistance training is low, injury does happen, and we have to apply certain principles to ensure that the risks are minimized.

Back

The fact that human beings stand upright in comparison to other animals provides a lot of benefits. We can see much further, and we are able to use our hands for other things while retaining an erect posture. This erectness has its own drawbacks, though the main one is that the discs in the spine become compressed. This compression takes place during walking, running, and sitting but also when we lift heavy loads. The back is prone to injury because it has to exert a force much larger than the object being lifted because it is so far from the ground. Back injuries are difficult to heal. They are quite painful, and it is difficult to do much else with a back injury; therefore, they really should be avoided during resistance training. The compressed discs in the lower back make it particularly vulnerable to injury. I am sure you have come across the age-old adage "lift with your legs, not with your back." Whenever you lift anything, you want to keep your back neutral so that your quads (legs) and core do most of the work and your back plays as small a role as possible in the execution of the movement. Your spine has an arch about it, and this position is much better than a rounded spine in carrying heavy loads. Arching that is extreme, however, increases the risk of a disk rupturing.

The Valsalva maneuver occurs when people are about to lift heavy and hold their breath to tighten their core. This maneuver can be dangerous for the heart because it creates a lot of pressure in the chest, and you can pass out. You will need to contract your core while breathing. The more you get stronger in your core, the easier this becomes. When weightlifting belts are used correctly, they can tighten the core enough to provide support such that the lift can be executed effectively. When used incorrectly, they can effectively weaken the core such that you won't be able to lift loads without a belt. Do not use a belt during exercises that do not require the lower back to work. When the lower back is engaged in an exercise, do not use a belt for light loads—use a belt when you are at maximal loads. A weightlifting belt supports heavy lifting, but it is by no means necessary for heavy lifting. If the core is trained properly, then it can become strong enough to support those loads.

Shoulders

The shoulder has a joint that is capable of rotation in any direction—it is the most mobile joint in the human body. This hyper-mobility is the reason why the shoulder is prone to injuries. The range of motion that the shoulder has can lead to structures acting on each other in undesirable ways. This can lead to tendonitis and inflammation. Ligaments, tendons, and muscles can be torn during high load resistance training. To prevent injury, you should warm up adequately and make sure that the shoulder is trained through all possible movements. This will keep the shoulder balanced.

Knees

The knee is located between two levers and separates the upper and lower legs. The main thing to look out for with regards to the knee is tendonitis. This tendonitis will occur when exercises are performed without following sound principles of progression. Too much intensity and volume too soon will result in tenderness and swelling. In yoga, the knee is prone to hyperextension; therefore, you are encouraged to keep the slightest bend in your knee. A lot of athletes use knee wraps, but the jury is still out on whether these actually prevent injury. Knee wraps support the extension of the knee but do not support knee stabilization as it has been purported. As with belts, their use should be limited to when you are working with the heaviest loads.

Elbows and Wrists

Wrists and elbows present the biggest risk of injury when loads are lifted overhead. The risk is less in exercises than in sports where there are a lot of overhead movements like tennis. When the elbow is overused, then it can dislocate. In gymnastics, as in yoga, the wrists are susceptible to injury, but in general, resistance training does not pose a huge threat to these joints.

Warm-Up

Warming up before exercise, including resistance training, is not optional—it is mandatory. The warm-up gets you in the right mental and physical state. The physiological effects of warm-ups can be divided into temperature-related and non-temperature-related effects. Muscle and core body temperature increase and improved neural function are some of the temperature-related effects, and increased flow of blood to the muscles and increased oxygen consumption are some of the non-temperature-related effects. Active or dynamic warm-ups are better than static ones. "The positive effects on performance many include the following: faster muscle contraction and relaxation of both agonist and antagonist muscles, improvements in the rate of force development and reaction time, improvements in muscle strength and power, lowered viscous resistance in muscles and joints, improved oxygen delivery, increased blood flow to active muscles, enhanced metabolic reactions and increased psychological preparedness for performance." (NSCA, 2015)

A warm-up consists of a general warm-up which will be about five minutes of slow aerobic movement such as walking on the treadmill, skipping, or cycling. The second part of the warm-up is the specific warm-up period which warms up the precise muscles you will target during the training session of about 10 minutes. Ian Jefferys came up with the best warm-up protocol using the acronym RAMP (Raise, Activate, Mobilize, Potentiate). Raise the temperature of the body and blood flow, activate the muscles you will be using, mobilize by practicing the movements you are going to be doing, and potentiate means to slowly increase the stress on the body (Jefferys, 2018).

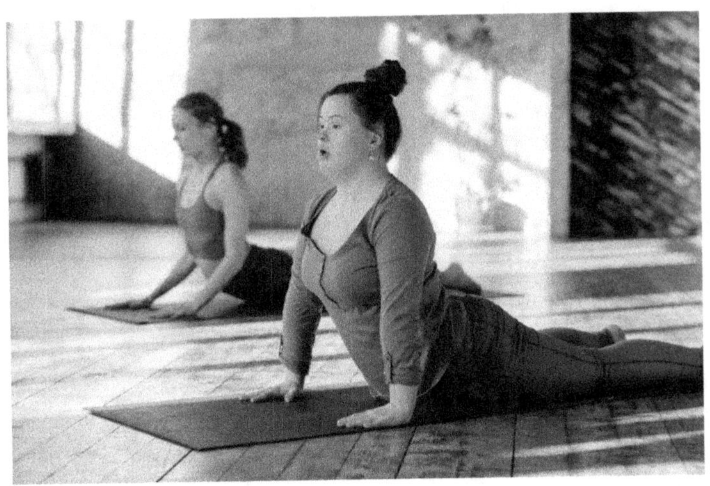

Cool Down

Andrew Huberman, a neuroscientist, released a skill acquisition podcast, and in there, he shared groundbreaking findings regarding learning a new skill. Usually, after an exercise session, we pick up our phones, hit the showers, or go grab a smoothie or coffee with a friend. Turns out that immediately turning to a different task is not the right move—we ineffectually leave gains on the table. Immediately after your workout, Huberman suggests we sit or lie still for about five minutes. There is a neurological process that takes place consolidating what we've just learned or practiced. We all know that we consolidate knowledge during sleep but we also consolidate immediately after the learning bout—as long as we give our minds the time. "There is also data showing that after any kind of motor movement provided, you're not bringing a lot more additional new sensory stimuli, there's a replay of the motor sequence that you performed correctly and there's an elimination of the motor sequences that you performed incorrectly, and they are run backwards in time." (Huberman, 2022)

Bad technique is eliminated, and the next time you practice the exercise, you perform it better. The yogis have known about this all along. They call it savasana. You lie down after a movement practice and integrate all the benefits that you have just tapped into. So after every exercise session, take five minutes in your car or locker room and immediately integrate it. Andy Galpin swears by this and calls it the anabolic window. Traditionally, the anabolic window is when you eat protein immediately after your workout to speed up and enhance protein synthesis, but Galpin sees it as a mental time. This is when you "Talk to your body, not listen to your body." Tell it that it is strong.

Cooldown is the part of the workout where you ease up on intensity or speed. It can take up to ten minutes. The cooldown lowers your heart rate. While you've been working out, your heart rate has been raised, and therefore you should cool down to make sure your blood pressure doesn't just drop precipitously and cause you dizziness and lightheadedness. This time can help you relax your mind, which I think I have described succinctly in the previous paragraph. Risks of injury are decreased as you cool down.

Stretch and make sure that your muscle fibers are elongated and able to take in the benefits of your workout. Delayed Onset Muscle Soreness (DOMS) is reduced. When your muscles get too sore after a workout, it can prevent you physically from being able to work out the next day or even discourage you mentally from training again. Your flexibility is also increased if your cool down is stretching. This will only make your strength training better as you are able to move your weight through larger ranges of motion. (Muthoni, 2021)

Program Design for Resistance Training

When it comes to designing an effective resistance training, you need to remember the principles from the beginning of the book. The acronym to bear in mind is SAID, which stands for Specific Adaptations to Imposed Demands. The type of demand you make on your body determines the adaptation. Your training program has to make use of overload, has to challenge your body, and cannot be what you are used to. The most available example is to gradually increase the load, but there are other ways to make use of this principle. You can increase the number of sessions per week (or per day for you superwomen out there), add more exercises, add more sets, switch up from simple to complex, or decrease the rest period between sets. Long-term training benefits are promoted through progression. You can increase your training intensity by increasing the number of weekly exercise sessions, adding more exercises, and changing the technical aspects of exercise. Make sure that your progression is structured and gradual. The following table lists the design variables that you need to incorporate into your program.

RESISTANCE TRAINING PROGRAM DESIGN VARIABLES
Needs analysis
Exercise selection
Training frequency
Exercise order
Training loads and repetitions
Volume
Rest periods

Resistance Training Across the Decades

Step 1: Needs Analysis

At the beginning of your journey, please consult your doctor to see if there is anything that you need to be aware of and any restrictions that need to be taken into consideration apart from the age factor.

If you have exercised before then this means that you are capable of much more than someone who has been sedentary. I have been in the fitness industry for seven years so my capabilities would be a bit different from some of you. Below is an example of classifying resistance exercise status.

RESISTANCE TRAINING BACKGROUND					
Status	Current program	Training Age	Frequency (per week)	Training Stress	Technique Experience and Skill
Beginner (untrained)	Not training	<2 months	< 3	None or low	None or minimal
Intermediate (moderately trained)	Currently trained	2-6 months	<4	Medium	Basic
Advanced (well trained)	Currently trained	> 1 year	>5	High	High

The primary goal for all of us is to improve our strength. That is the adaptation we are seeking, and we should focus on that.

Step 2: Exercise Selection

Now we move to choosing the exercises that will make us stronger. There are hundreds of resistance training exercises we can choose from, but our driver is understanding which muscle groups we want to target. We'll have core exercises (large muscle group, multi-joints) and assistance exercises (single joint, smaller muscle groups). Assistance exercises are also used in injury prevention. As you get older, you will be using a lot more assistance exercises. We need to make sure that we have muscle balance as well and that we do not favor certain muscle groups and neglect others. Weaknesses have to be addressed and worked on to ensure that the body is balanced. If you are starting out, then start with machines to learn the technique and use weight-assisted exercises. The core and assistance exercises are listed in the following table.

EXERCISE SELECTION	
Core	**Assistance**
Flat bench press with dumbbell/barbell (chest)	Flat fly dumbbells (chest)
Incline bench press with barbell/dumbbell (chest)	Incline fly dumbbells (chest)
Machine bench press flat/incline/decline (chest)	Cable crossover standing (chest)
Lat pulldown (back)	Incline bench cable crossover (chest)
90-degree machine row (back)	Stiff leg deadlifts (back)
Chin up (back)	Barbell good mornings (back)
One arm row with dumbbell (back)	Lower back extension (back)
Machine row (back)	Lying back extension (back)
T bar row (back)	Leg extension (legs)
Straight arm pulldown (back)	Lying leg curl (legs)
Straight arm pullover (back)	Seated calf raises (legs)

One arm cable pulldown (back)	Standing calf raises (legs)
Dumbbell straight arm pullback (back)	Lateral raises with dumbbells (shoulders)
Squats with barbell (legs)	Front raises (shoulders)
Lunges with barbell (legs)	Bent over lateral raises (shoulders)
45-degree leg press (legs)	Dumbbell or barbell standing curl (biceps)
Hack squat (legs)	Seated dumbbell curl (biceps)
Step ups (legs)	Preacher curls (biceps)
Deadlifts (legs)	Hammer curls (biceps)
Dips (triceps)	Reverse grip barbell curls (biceps)
	Triceps push down (triceps)
	Overhead cable extension (triceps)
	French press (triceps)
	Kickback with dumbbells (triceps)

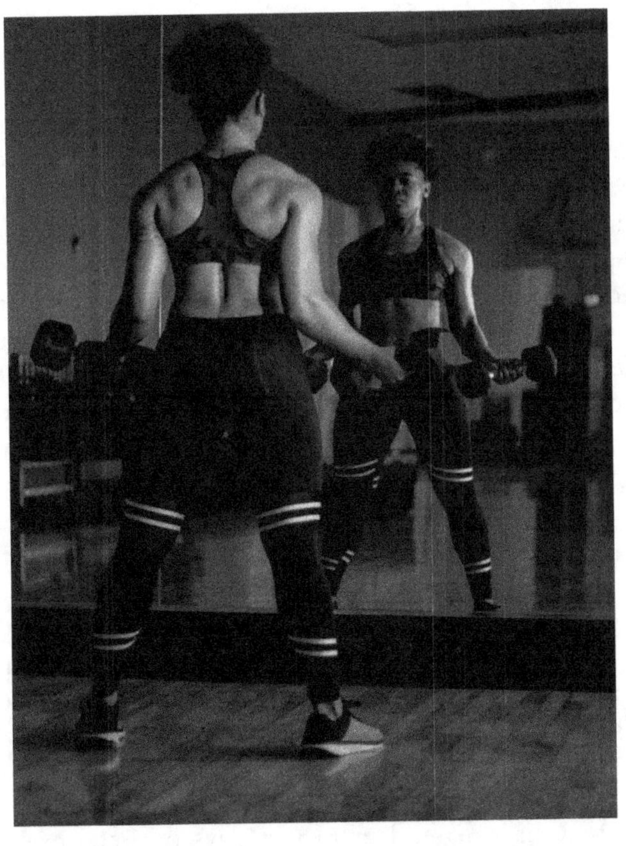

It's important that you factor in how much time you have to work out. Women from their twenties to fifties may have a lot less time than older women. Some exercises take much longer to perform than others, so the ones that are time efficient would need to be prioritized over the ones that take longer. A machine is usually easier than free weights, which need to be arranged and stacked, locked on both sides.

Step 3: Training Frequency

The training frequency is the measure of the number of exercise sessions within a given period. We will use one week as our period. There is a model called the Fitness-fatigue model, which is used to determine your preparedness (capacity) for your next workout. "According to the fitness-fatigue model, at any time preparedness is the difference between the positive effects of fitness and the negative effects of fatigue. But since fatigue, although very great, doesn't stick around very long we can take advantage of the fitness gained without over-training. Intuitively it has to be this way or you'd never have any apparent progress. What it really means is that it allows us to take advantage of the fact that while the fatigue impulse may be twice as high as the fitness impulse, the fatigue decays three times as fast. The fitness gained is still a result of the training impulse. This is a simplified explanation of the fitness-fatigue model." (Troy, 2018)

As you get older, your preparedness may decrease, and you may have to add extra rest days between exercise sessions. For most of us, three days a week of exercise sessions are enough. The number of exercise sessions can be increased as you get stronger. The general rule is to have at least one full recovery day a week but not more than three. Space out your workouts in the week. If you have three workouts, then use Monday, Wednesday, and Friday. If you exercise on Monday, Tuesday, and Wednesday, by the time Monday comes again, you will have lost all the gains you've made. The following is a guideline for training frequency.

<table>
<tr><td colspan="2">RESISTANCE TRAINING FREQUENCY BASED ON TRAINING STATUS</td></tr>
<tr><td>Training Status</td><td>Frequency Guidelines</td></tr>
<tr><td>Beginner</td><td>2-3</td></tr>
<tr><td>Intermediate</td><td>3-4</td></tr>
<tr><td>Advanced</td><td>4-7</td></tr>
</table>

As you get more comfortable with resistance training, you can use a split routine where you train different muscle groups on different days, allowing the ones that are not to be exercised to recover. So one day, you may workout legs, then work out your shoulders and back the next day. Alternating between the upper and lower body is a great way to work out most days. Here are examples of common split routines for you to use as guidelines.

Training Day	Body Parts	Sun	Mon	Tues	Wed
1	Lower body	Rest	Lower body	Upper body	Rest
2	Upper body				
1	Chest, shoulders, triceps	Rest	Chest shoulders, triceps	Lower body	Back, traps, biceps
2	Lower body				

3	Back, trapezius, biceps				
1	Chest, and back	Chest and back	Lower body	Shoulders and arms	Rest
2	Lower body				
3	Shoulders and arms				
Thur	**Fri**	**Sat**			
Lower body	Upper body	Rest			
Rest	Chest, shoulders, triceps	Lower body			
Chest and back	Lower body	Shoulder and arms			

If your occupation is one that keeps you on your feet all day long, then you may not be able to have a lot of training sessions.

Step 4: Exercise Order

"Exercise order refers to a sequence of resistance exercises performed during one training session. Although there are many ways to arrange exercises, decisions are invariably based on how one exercise affects the quality of effort of the technique of another exercise." (NSCA, 2015)

There are different ways for you to plan your program.

Power-Other Core-Assistance:

You want to start with the most demanding exercises that require the most concentration and the highest skill, then move to other core exercises that aren't power output-driven, then finish off with assistance exercises. When you are tired, it's hard to execute difficult exercises while maintaining good form. This could result in an injury.

Alternate Between Upper and Lower Body Exercises:

If you are still new at resistance training, then this may be the better option for you. You are probably not doing intense power core exercises such as snatches. Not yet anyway. You may also not be able to do consecutive upper body movements one after the other; therefore, you should alternate between the upper and lower body. This could also result in an exercise session that takes a shorter time to complete.

Alternate between Push and Pull Exercises:

Alternate between exercises that require you to push (shoulder press, tricep extensions, and bench press) and those that require you to pull (bent-over row, biceps curl, and lat. pulldown). This will improve your recovery and allow you to have the capacity to recruit all the muscles needed to complete your exercise session. The same muscle groups will not be used in a sequence, reducing fatigue. The lower body has push and pull exercises as well. When you push against the floor, it's a pushing movement, squats would be an example of this, and a leg curl would be a pull exercise.

Supersets and Compound Sets:

A superset is when you perform two exercises one after the other with no rest in between. They would stimulate two opposing muscle areas. For example, you would start with biceps curls and then move into tricep extensions. A compound set is performing two consecutive movements with little or no rest on muscles in the same group. You may complete ten bicep curls, then move on to hammer curls. Supersets and compound sets are time efficient but are also quite demanding on your body; therefore, newbies should not be doing these. The more advanced of you should definitely incorporate these into your sessions.

Step 5: Training Loads and Repetitions

The most critical part of resistance training is the resistance, i.e., the load. This is the amount of weight that you use in a set. There is an inverse relationship between the number of reps you are able to perform and the load. When the load increases, the reps decrease, and vice versa, which is why load is usually measured in terms of your maximum load capability. Basically, when you choose your load and your repetitions, but you realize that you could have gone for five more reps, then you chose a load that was too light. Your last repetition in a set should be a tough time. There are loads where you can only do one repetition at that weight. That is your maximum, and it's 100% (RM). A guideline is provided to you to figure out how many reps you should aim for at a given weight.

%1RM	Number of Reps
100	1
95	2
93	3
90	4
87	5
85	6
83	7
80	8
77	9
75	10
70	11
67	12
65	15

If you are performing more than one set (recommended), then you will need to decrease the load in order to maintain the number of repetitions, or you will need to decrease the reps to maintain the load. You will be able to do more work on a machine than with free weights. The larger the muscle groups, the more reps you can perform in general, and smaller muscle groups require less reps. The best way for you to determine your 1RM is to use the conversion chart I have included. Choose a weight and see how many reps you can perform until you are unable to, then the table will tell you how much your maximum is.

RM	1	2	3	4	5	6
% 1RM	100	95	93	90	87	85
Load (kg or lbs)	10	10	9	9	9	9
	20	19	19	18	17	17
	30	29	28	27	26	26
	40	38	37	36	35	34
	50	48	47	45	44	43
	60	57	56	54	52	51
	70	67	65	63	6	60
	80	76	74	72	70	68
	90	86	84	81	78	77
	100	95	93	90	87	85

7	8	9	10	12	15
83	80	77	75	67	65
8	8	8	8	7	7
17	16	15	15	13	3
25	24	23	23	20	20
33	32	31	30	27	26
43	40	39	38	34	33
50	48	46	45	40	39
58	56	54	53	47	46
66	64	62	60	54	52
75	72	69	68	60	59
83	80	77	75	67	65

Since our training goal is strength, you are looking at no more than six repetitions for a load that is equal to or more than 85% of 1RM. The next question that you would ask is how do I know when to increase my load and progress? The easiest rule to remember for this is the 2-for-2-rule. If you can execute two more reps in a set in two consecutive workouts. then you can increase your load. The next table gives you an idea of how much load you can increase your progressions with.

LOAD INCREASES		
Description	**Body Area Exercise**	**Estimated Load Increases**
Smaller, weaker, less trained	Upper body	2.5-5 lbs (1-2 kg)
	Lower body	5-10 lbs (2-4 kg)
Larger, stronger, more trained	Upper body	5-10+lbs (2-4+ kg)
	Lower body	10-15+lbs (4-7+ kg)

Step 6: Volume

Volume is the number of sets that you perform in an exercise session. If you are really new to resistance training, then one set would work, but in general, you need much more volume in order to adapt your body for strength. In at least one of your sets, you need to reach failure and the other sets have to be near failure for you to become stronger. Remember that you have to overload your body, or else you will not make gains. For strength, the number of sets you should aim for is between two and six.

Step 7: Rest Periods

The rest period is the time you are waiting in between sets. The rest for beginners will be a bit more on the longer side. The amount of rest is related to the amount of load that you are working with. The higher the load, the higher the rest. For strength, we will rest 2-5 min between sets. As you get stronger and more proficient, you will be easing to 2 minutes. The older of you may need to spend more time resting.

Conclusion

I think after reading this, you agree that skinny is the new strong. You have been given everything you need for the new journey you are about to embark on. We've busted some myths and have seen strength in a very different way. We have gone "underneath the hood" and taken time to understand our bodies in greater detail so that we have a clearer understanding of how all our hard work will benefit us. We understand why everything we will do from now onwards is determined by us and what we tell ourselves. I hope your confidence is soaring, and even when things get difficult, you are still self-efficacious.

Have a healthy relationship with food. Do not get wrapped up in Not Rules. Don't eat this, don't eat that. Don't see food as forbidden. See it as empowering. Eat food that empowers you to do all the things you want to do, that makes you make the most of your time, and remember variety is the spice for your body. Most importantly. Eat!

Breathe! Use your diaphragm and use your fitness as a way to relax. It does not have to be another chore—this is when you can savor your life. Any fitness journey incorporates sufficient rest and recovery. Show up to your workouts with intention and gusto. Tap into your mind-body connection.

Get Strong!

Be Strong!

Live strong!

And finish life strong!

References

Alexander, A. (2021). *The align method : 5 movement principles for a stronger body, sharper mind, and stress-proof life*. Grand Central Publishing.

August 2020, I. W.-L. S. C. 23. (2020). *Does your personality change as you get older?* Livescience.com. https://www.livescience.com/personality-age-change.html

Bandura, A. (1977). *Self-efficacy: toward a Unifying Theory of Behavioral Change.* Psycnet.apa.org. https://psycnet.apa.org/record/1977-25733-001

Brennan, D. (2021, November 27). *What Is Proprioception?* WebMD. https://www.webmd.com/brain/what-is-proprioception

DK. (2009). *Strength training : the complete step-by-step guide to a stronger, sculpted body*. Penguin Random House.

Ericsson, A. (2017). *Peak*. Vintage.

Gordillo, F., Mestas, L., Arana, J. M., Pérez, M. Á., & Escotto, E. A. (2017). The Effect of Mortality Salience and Type of Life on Personality Evaluation. *Europe's Journal of Psychology, 13*(2), 286–299. https://doi.org/10.5964/ejop.v13i2.1149

Holmes, T. (2017, April 11). *Macrocycles, Mesocycles and Microcycles: Understanding the 3 Cycles of Periodization.* TrainingPeaks.
https://www.trainingpeaks.com/blog/macrocycles-mesocycles-and-microcycles-understanding-the-3-cycles-of-periodization/

Huberman, A. (2021, May 17). *How to Learn Skills Faster | Huberman Lab Podcast #20.* YouTube.
https://www.youtube.com/watch?v=xJ0IBzCjEPk&ab_channel=AndrewHuberman

Hurrell, R. F., & Finot, P. A. (1990). *The Maillard Reaction in Food Processing, Human Nutrition and Physiology.* Birkhauser.

Jefferys, I. (2018). *(PDF) Jeffreys I (2007) Warm-up revisited: The ramp method of optimizing warm-ups. Professional Strength and Conditioning. (6) 12-18.* ResearchGate.
https://www.researchgate.net/publication/280945961_Jeffreys_I_2007_Warm-up_revisited_The_ramp_method_of_optimizing_warm-ups_Professional_Strength_and_Conditioning_6_12-18

Jonas. (2021, July 21). *Importance of Cooling Down After Exercise - jonas Muthoni.* Www.jonasmuthoni.com.
https://jonasmuthoni.com/blog/importance-cooling-down-post-exercise/#:~:text=Reduces%20DOMS%20(Delayed%20Onset%20Muscle%20Soreness)&text=This%20indicates%20that%20cooling%20down

Kersting, K. (2003). Personality changes for the better with age. *APA* https://www.apa.org/monitor/julaug03/personality

Kotler, S. (2022). *Frequently Asked Questions on Flow - Steven Kotler.* Steven Kotler. https://www.stevenkotler.com/rabbit-hole/frequently-asked-questions-on-flow

Mc Clelland, D. C. (1953). *APA PsycNet.* Psycnet.apa.org. https://psycnet.apa.org/record/2006-09558-000

Nestor, J. (2020). *Breath : the new science of a lost art.* Riverhead Books.

NIH. (2022, June 14). *NIA Strategic Directions 2020-2025.* National Institute on Aging. https://www.nia.nih.gov/about/aging-strategic-directions-research

NSCA. (2015). *Essentials of Strength Training and Conditioning.* Human Kinetics.

Paul Morris Fitts, & Posner, M. I. (1967). *Human performance.* Greenwood Press.

Payne, A. (2022). *Body Types: How to Train & Diet for Your Body Type.* Blog.nasm.org. https://blog.nasm.org/fitness/body-types-how-to-train-diet-for-your-body-type

Perera, A. (2021, June 10). *Framing Effect | Simply Psychology.* Www.simplypsychology.org.

https://www.simplypsychology.org/framing-effect.html

Robbins, T. (2017). *Goal Setting is the Secret to a Compelling Future.* Tonyrobbins.com. https://www.tonyrobbins.com/ask-tony/can-create-compelling-future/

Robson, D. (2006, March 12). *The Importance Of The Pump: Anthony Catanzaro Is Here To Pump You Up!* Bodybuilding.com. https://www.bodybuilding.com/content/the-importance-of-the-pump-anthony-cantanzaro-is-here-to-pump-you-up.html#:~:text=One%20bodybuilder%20who%20has%20pumped

Ronnberg, O. (2017). *Strength Training for Women.* Skyhorse.

September 3, L. B. W.-R., & 2020. (2020, September 3). *The Best Foods to Eat in Your 20s, 30s, 40s, and 50s.* Eat This Not That. https://www.eatthis.com/best-foods-for-every-decade/

Stanfield, J. (2019, May 14). *Fitness for Every Decade: What Every Woman Should Know.* ACE. https://www.acefitness.org//resources/everyone/blog/7290/fitness-for-every-decade-what-every-woman-should-know/